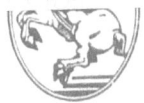

Gerhard Kletter

The Extra-Intracranial Bypass Operation for Prevention and Treatment of Stroke

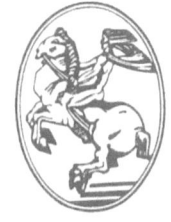

Springer-Verlag Wien GmbH

Dr. GERHARD KLETTER
Department of Neurosurgery (Head: Prof. Dr. W. TH. KOOS),
University of Vienna Medical School, Vienna, Austria

With 105 Figures

© 1979 by Springer-Verlag Wien

Originally published by Springer Vienna in 1979.

ISBN 978-3-7091-2060-6   ISBN 978-3-7091-2058-3 (eBook)
DOI 10.1007/978-3-7091-2058-3

Library of Congress Cataloging in Publication Data. Kletter, Gerhard, 1942-   . The
extra-intracranial bypass operation for prevention and treatment of stroke. Includes
bibliographical references and index. 1. Cerebrovascular disease—Surgery. 2. Cerebral
arteries—Surgery. 3. Microsurgery. I. Title. [DNLM: 1. Cerebrovascular disorders—Surgery. 2. Cerebrovascular disorders—Prevention and control. 3. Arteries—Surgery. 4.
Cerebral arteries—Surgery. WL 335.3. K 64 e] RD 594.2. K 58. 617′.481. 79-3989.

To
Shebby

Foreword

A decade has passed since systematic studies were initiated in the USA in an attempt at establishing the experimental basis for a surgical technique which was to prove an effective tool in combatting one of the most common diseases, i.e. cerebrovascular accidents. The development of such intricate vasculosurgical techniques as are required for extra-intracranial arterial bypass operations would not have been possible without the aid of the surgical microscope, which had been designed some years earlier. In the past few years increasing emphasis has been placed on establishing clear-cut indications for the bypass operation, because satisfactory long-term results are unlikely to be obtained without them. Needless to say that this requires a close cooperation of the neurosurgeon with a team composed of neurologists, internists, radiologists, and pathologists. Fortunately enough, cooperation between the services of the University of Vienna Medical School proved to be exemplary.

While there has been no lack of efforts by major medical centers both in Europe and the overseas countries to perfect bypass operations for cerebrovascular accidents, a comprehensive monograph reviewing all medical and operative problems involved in microvascular surgery for strokes was badly missed by many.

Thus the present book by my collaborator Dr. Kletter no doubt fills a gap in the medical literature on this subject. Conceived to account for what has been experienced as a definite need by clinicians, the monograph offers an excellent review of microsurgical alternatives in the operative management of cerebrovascular lesions. At the same time the author explicitly outlines the indications of extra-intracranial bypass operations with due reference to the patient's overall condition. Experimental studies in vascular pathology and vascular surgery conducted by him proved to be of fundamental importance for the success of surgery.

For all of these reasons it is to be hoped that the present book will find a large readership.

Vienna, March 1979 *Wolfgang Th. Koos*

Preface

To begin with, I should like to express my deep gratitude to my superior, Prof. Dr. med. Wolfgang Koos, without whose encouragement this work would never have been embarked upon. It was he, in fact, who aroused my interest in, and fostered my enthusiasm for, vascular neurosurgery. At his instigation I was given the opportunity of spending one year at the Neurosurgery Service in Zurich, working first with Professor Krayenbühl and subsequently with Professor Yaşargil.

I am indebted to Professors Yaşargil and Yonekawa for the operative technique, detailed in this book, which I had the good fortune of learning from them.

In acquiring the basic morphologic knowledge needed for this operative technique I was guided by Professor Holzner from the Department of Pathologic Anatomy, University of Vienna Medical School.

My thanks are also tendered to Professor Reisner, medical director of the Neurology Department, University of Vienna Medical School, who granted me access to data on computer tomography, cerebral blood flow measurements and scintigraphy without which this work would not have been complete.

For the experimental studies conducted in Vienna I am under special obligation to Professor Gottlob, in charge of the Department of Experimental Surgery, who offered me generous assistance and much invaluable advice.

To Dr. Meyermann I wish to present my thanks for the most fruitful cooperation from which I have benefited ever since we worked together in Zurich.

Dr. Schuster, my colleague at the Neurosurgery Department, has been of invaluable help in following up on the progress of our patients and condensing the material into scientific data.

My thanks are also due to Dr. Adelheid Flohr for typing the manuscript, to Ms. Maria Mayer who gave me a helping hand with the tables and graphs, and to Dr. Christa Körbler who read the galley proofs.

Last, but assuredly not least, I should like to express my sincere appreciation to the publishers, first and foremost Dr. W. Schwabl, and secondly to his staff at Springer-Verlag, who have spared no effort in assuring the speedy publication of this book.

Vienna, March 1979   *Gerhard Kletter*

Contents

Abbreviations

AN, ANA	Anastomosis
BICO	Bilateral internal carotid occlusion
CA	Carotid artery
CAT, CT	Computerized (axial) tomography
CBF	Cerebral blood flow
CS	Completed stroke
CV	Cortical vessel
EIAB	Extra-intracranial arterial bypass
GLPS	Generalized low perfusion syndrome
ICA	Internal carotid artery
ICO	Internal carotid artery occlusion
Kr^{84}	Krypton
MCA	Middle cerebral artery
MCO	Middle cerebral artery occlusion
OA	Occipital artery
PRIND	Prolonged reversible ischemic neurological deficit
PS	Progressive stroke
rCBF	Regional cerebral blood flow
RIND	Reversible ischemic neurological deficit
SC	Spinal cord
SEP	Stimulated evoked potentials
STA	Superficial temporal artery
Tc^{99}	Technetium
TIA	Transient ischemic attack
VA	Vertebral artery
WHO	World Health Organization
Xe^{133}	Xenon

1. Introduction

Since the first extra-intracranial bypass operation was performed by Yaşargil in 1967, a great number of studies dealing with this surgical technique have been published. Quite naturally, this method was viewed with great scepticism in the first years following its introduction. The first clinical results showed surprising success, particularly in transient ischemic attacks and in mild forms of completed stroke. At the beginning, this success was merely accepted as an empirical fact; the theoretical foundations of this operative technique were worked out only gradually. Although comprehensive studies on this subject have already been published, they all were written by several authors as a congress report and are thus necessarily repetitive. It is hard to use these publications as a guideline for this new operation. Neurosurgeons not yet familiar with the problems associated with this technique, and particularly with the indications for such surgery, will find it difficult to decide, in view of the great number of publications available and the diverging opinions they express, which study is applicable to their particular situation.

The present study is an attempt to integrate the data available. For this reason, it starts with a short historical survey, followed by a very concise discussion of the epidemiology of stroke, and then deals with the most essential anatomical data. Particular attention is paid to the pathology of the superficial temporal artery, as it became evident after the introduction of this surgical technique that this operation is made possible only by the specific pathological and anatomical characteristics of this vessel.

As these characteristics must also be taken into account during the operation, the chapter about pathophysiology is elaborated upon in greater detail, in order to provide a better understanding of the technique and the results achieved.

The method itself is described as it is practiced at the Department of Neurosurgery, Vienna, although other common techniques, which, by the way, do not differ very much, are also discussed.

Much attention is also paid to preoperative diagnostics and the evaluation of the indication for extra-intracranial anastomosis. For the first time, an attempt is made to distinguish the examinations that are essential for the various types of indication. This approach is based on the consideration that not all the neurosurgical hospitals in which extra-intracranial anastomosis can be quite easily performed as far as the technique is concerned have all the commonly used examination methods at their disposal.

The results of surgery done at the Department of Neurosurgery in Vienna, which are mor or less identical to those obtained at other neurosurgical centers, are reported. In addition, statistical data from the other centers are used in order to permit a better evaluation of the technique. These statistics also include patients who had surgery than 10 years ago. It is true that this follow-up period, and even a shorter one, as found in many instances, do not permit a judgment as to whether this operative method can decisively improve the long-term mobidity rate of stroke. However, at present the incorporation of a very large number of patients, whose cases extend over longer periods of time, into one study is being attempted (cooperative study of Barnett and Peerless).

On the present study a firm stand is taken in regard to certain controversial issues. Although these evaluations may eventually prove to be partly incorrect, definite statements are sometimes necessary in order to provoke criticism and thus lead to new findings.

This publication will have achieved its objective if it provides a guideline to surgeons not familiar with this new operative method, and if those who have already dealt with this technique will be induced to reconsider their own views, as well as those expressed in this study, with a critical eye.

2. A Historical Survey of Extra-Intracranial Anastomosis

The possible occlusion of the internal carotid artery or its branches has been known for centuries. As far back as 1684, Sir Thomas Willis described such an occlusion, and in 1818, Abercrombie reported a carotid occlusion associated with a cerebral focus. Cohnheim (1872) and Wernicke (1881) assumed that intracerebral changes were caused by occlusions or stenoses of the large afferent arteries. It was not until 1905 that a systematic pathological study of carotid occlusions was published (Chiari 1905). During the following decades, these findings were further supported by additional research work, but surgery was out of the question for lack of technical means. Therefore no measures could be taken to prevent an imminent stroke by eliminating a stenosis in the large afferent vessels. Due to insufficient knowledge in regard to the pathophysiology and pathogenesis of cerebral vascular occlusions and their symptoms, incorrect methods were adopted. For example, in selected cases a section of the stenosed carotid vessel was completely ligated to prevent embolism in cerebral vessels.

The first carotid endarterectomies were performed in 1953 (Cooley 1954, De Bakey 1964, 1965). As the indications for surgery became more well-defined, better and better results were obtained (Dorndorf 1965). However, as reconstructive vascular surgery was applied to the large arteries of the head to an increasing extent, it became evident that these surgical procedures were not feasible in all cases of vascular changes leading or having led to a stroke. About 90 percent of all cerebral infarction is due to an occlusion or a stenosis of one or several afferent cerebral vessels. Two-thirds of these changes are found extracranially, and one-third intracranially. For technical reasons, a surgical approach was not practicable for all extracranial changes (*e.g.*, carotid occlusions).

Thus surgery was not feasible in 30 to 40 percent of all stroke cases (Acheson 1964, Melamed 1973, WHO 1975), which led to a rather unsatisfactory situation. Approximately two-thirds of the patients who had had a stroke, or in whom a stroke was imminent, could undergo successful surgical treatment. For the remaining one-third, however, there was no surgical treatment better than that available at the beginning of this century. Numerous authors tried to approach the occluded intracranial cerebral vessels directly (Welch 1956, Scheibert 1959, Jacobson *et al.* 1960, Shillito 1961, Chou 1963, Lougheed 1963, Woringer and Kunlin 1963, Yaşargil 1969).

However, due to technical problems associated with this direct method, it was not generally adopted. Fisher (1951), pointing out this unsatisfactory situation, suggested that surgeons "should study the practicability of linking extra- and intracranial circulation". Ten years later, this view was again strongly supported by Walls at the Princetown Conference on Cerebral Vascular Disease.

At that time, these ideas by Fisher and Walls could not be implemented for technical reasons. Although anastomosis of small vessels and the vascular suture technique, as well as the technique of organ transplantation, were described by Carell and Gouthrie in 1912, it was not until the introduction of the operating microscope that vessels so minute as the superficial temporal artery and the middle cerebral artery could be successfully anastomosed. Microvascular surgery was first performed by Jacobson and Suarez in 1960. A few years later this technique was refined by Buncke and Schultz (1965) and was then introduced into plastic surgery. Thus the means necessary for putting already existing ideas into practice became available.

Experimental models were developed by Donaghy and Yaşargil (1967), and extra-intracranial anastomosis between the superficial temporal artery and the middle cerebral artery was performed for the first time by each of the two authors in Zurich and Vermont, respectively, on June 7, 1967. Yaşargil performed two further operations on August 14 and 22, 1967 (Krayenbühl and Yaşargil 1968).

As was the case when surgery was first performed on extracranial vessels, it took a long time to find out in which cases this new technique was indicated. In 1969, Yaşargil compared the results of nine operations of this kind with the results of direct embolectomy of the middle cerebral artery. His findings spoke clearly in favor of extra-intracranial anastomosis. This new surgical technique found wide application only gradually. In 1969, Matsubara reported one case in which this method was used. In 1971, 44 cases were presented in Prague by their respective authors. In 60 percent of the patients, neurological symptoms had definitely improved. At the First Symposium on Microvascular Anastomosis in Loma Linda, California, 301 cases were presented by 25 neurosurgeons. At the Second Symposium in 1974, more than 450 patients had already undergone extra-intracranial anastomosis.

During the past 2 years, this operative method has found such wide acceptance that the exact number of patients who have been operated on can no longer be precisely ascertained. Neurosurgeons using this technique have reported initial results of 100 such operations and results in patients monitored postoperatively over a sufficient period of time (Chater and Popp 1976, Gratzl et al. 1976, Yonekawa and Yaşargil 1976). At present, the number of extra-intracranial anastomoses performed all over the world probably totals between 15,000 and 20,000.

3. Epidemiology of Stroke

In all industrial and developed countries, diseases of the cerebral vessels rank third among the causes of death. The classification of cerebrovascular diseases as shown in Table 1 has proven to be of clinical value. The incidence rate is based on the work of Kurtzke (1969), who analyzed the results of field studies carried out in the United States and Australia.

Table 1 demonstrates the frequency of cerebral embolism and thrombosis. In the United States, approximately 400,000 new strokes occur each year (0,2 percent of the population), of which 80 percent are due to cerebrovascular occlusive diseases (Whisnant *et al*. 1973). The rate of incidence in the other Western industrial countries is almost as high. Only 5 to 15 percent of new strokes are due to subarachnoid hemorrhage, a major area of interest to the neurosurgeon. A mortality rate of between 21 and 35 percent has been descriebed by various authors (Reisner *et al*. 1973). This rate refers to deaths occurring in the first 6 months following a stroke of sclerotic origin. Within 24 months, the death rate decreases gradually and finally corresponds to that of the overall population of the same age group. Some authors mentioned a much higher mortality rate. Dorndorf (1968), for example, observed a mortality rate of 54 percent during the first 6 months after stroke.

Other publications also mention geographical, racial, and genetic variations, but going into these details would exceed the scope of this chapter.

Table 1. *The Frequency of Cerebrovascular Lesions*

1.	Ischemic attack (cerebral embolism and thrombosis)	63%
2.	Cerebral hemorrhage	15%
3.	Subarachnoid hemorrhage	12%
4.	Other vascular lesions in the CNS	10%

In recent years, the average age of stroke victims has shifted downward (Dorndorf 1969, Brenner and Kletter 1978, Reisner *et al*. 1961, 1965, 1968, 1971, 1973). In 1958, Lindgren reported an average age of 52.7 years, Dorndorf, in 1968, 49.1 years, and Marshall, in 1971, 51 years. These data emphasize the fact that two-thirds of all stroke patients are under 65, an age group consisting of people who are still employed.

Environmental factors and a higher and a higher life expectancy account for a notable increase in stroke incidence over the past 10 to 15 years.

Once a stroke has occurred, rehabilitation is extremely difficult (Gordon and Kohn 1966, Peszlynski *et al.* 1972, Wahle 1975); thus it is preferable to perform surgery at the stage of transient ischemic attacks (TIA), which very often precede the stroke. Statistical studies have shown that there is an 18 to 60 percent probability that patients suffering from TIA will have a completed stroke within 1 year (Marshal 1971).

Thus surgical procedures must, above all, aim at preventing an imminent stroke. After a stroke, however, they should be applied to improve the quality of life. In the preceding chapter it was mentioned that two-thirds of occlusive or stenosing processes are located extra-cranially; these accounts, for 40 percent of all cerebrovascular diseases. In the remaining 20 percent a surgical approach by means of extra-intracranial anastomosis is applicable. This operation aims either at preventing the stroke, or at least partly improving the patient's condition after a clinically operable stroke. Thus the quality of life may be enhanced, and in certain cases almost complete rehabilitation may be achieved.

4. Anatomy and Pathophysiology

4.1. The Superficial Temporal Artery

The external carotid artery bifurcates in the area between the ear and the temporomandibular joint into the internal maxillary artery on one side, and into the superficial temporal artery on the other side. After giving off a branch (the transverse facial artery) the superficial temporal artery crosses the zygomatic arch and then becomes palpable. It then ascends along the temporal fascia and divides into a rather large parietal ramus and a rather thin anterior ramus, which nourish the anterior and middle areas of the galea (Fig. 1). Histologically, it is a muscular-type artery with an average trunk diameter of approximately 0,6 cm. As do other arteries of the same caliber, this vessel has an intima, an elastica interna, a media, and a relatively large adventitia.

For extra-intracranial anastomosis the integrity and the structure of the afferent vessel—in this case the superficial temporal artery—are of paramount importance. As the surgical procedure described in the present study is generally used in patients showing rather severe generalized arteriosclerosis, it is essential to clarify the changes that this vessel undergoes in old age or in severe generalized arteriosclerosis. The problem of blood flow must also be considered, because at the site generally used for anastomosis this vessel has an average lumen diameter of 1.2 to 1.5 mm, a caliber that can barely replace the internal carotid.

Before it was used in extra-intracranial anastomosis little attention was paid to the superficial temporal artery. Changes in it caused by senility, course variations, and degenerative transformations were of no substantial interest in clinical practice. A report on this artery was first published by Henschen (1950), who placed a flap of the temporal muscle onto an ischemic cortex area, thereby causing the neurological symptoms to decrease after a few days. Before extra-intracranial bypass was introduced, only Ainsworth et al. (1961) and Lie et al. (1970) had conducted major studies dealing with this vessel. In about 30 percent of all cases Lie found calcifications that were mostly perivascular and mild.

To elucidate the qualitative changes involved, this author carried out histopathological and physiological studies involving the superficial temporal artery in more than 200 routine cases of both sexes and different age groups at the Department of Pathology, University of Vienna (Head: Prof. Dr. J. H. Holzner). The left temporal artery was removed just before it bifurcates into its two main branches. This site was considered histologically representative. Comparable ipsilateral sections

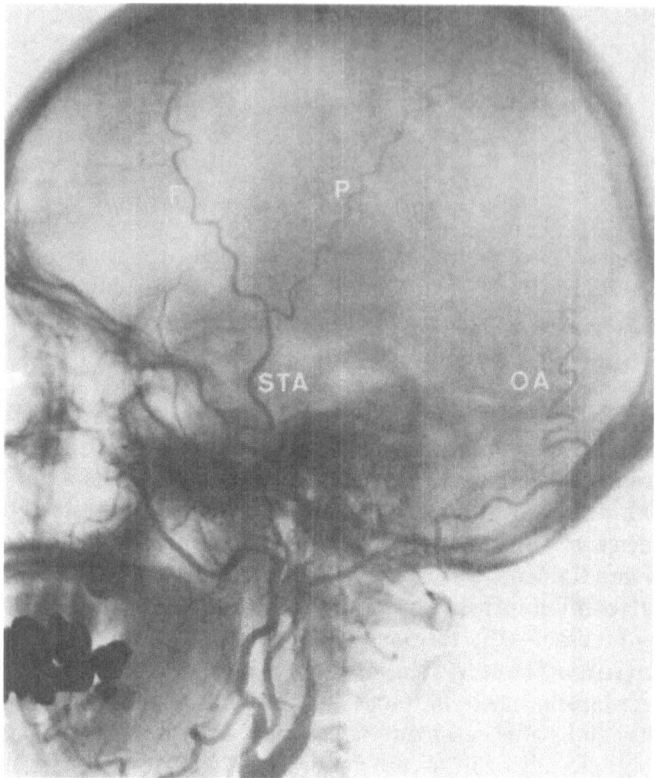

Fig. 1. Angiogram of the external carotid artery and the extracranial vessels used in extra-intracranial anastomosis. Note the superficial temporal artery (*STA*) with its parietal (*P*) and frontal (*F*) branches and the occipital artery (*OA*)

of the carotid bifurcation, the siphon part of the internal carotid artery, and the middle cerebral artery were taken and examined histologically in 50 cases. On addition a small portion of the superficial temporal artery was examined histologically in nearly all the patients who underwent extra-intracranial bypass operation at the Department of Neurosurgery, Vienna. The histological sections were stained with hematoxylin-eosin, van Gieson, Elastica, Kossa-Pas, and Alzian (Kletter *et al.* 1975, 1976).

The most significant morphological finding in this material was a progressive narrowing of the lumen. This effect was due to proliferation associated with senile enlargement of the superficial temporal artery. It seems of particular importance that no large calcium deposits were found. In only 3 of more than 300 sections were there slight calcerous changes (Figs. 2 and 3). In reality, sclerotic changes in the superficial temporal artery progress at the same rate as in other vessels of the human body. In comparison with other vessels there is hardly any difference in the degree of arteriosclerosis. The observed difference lies in

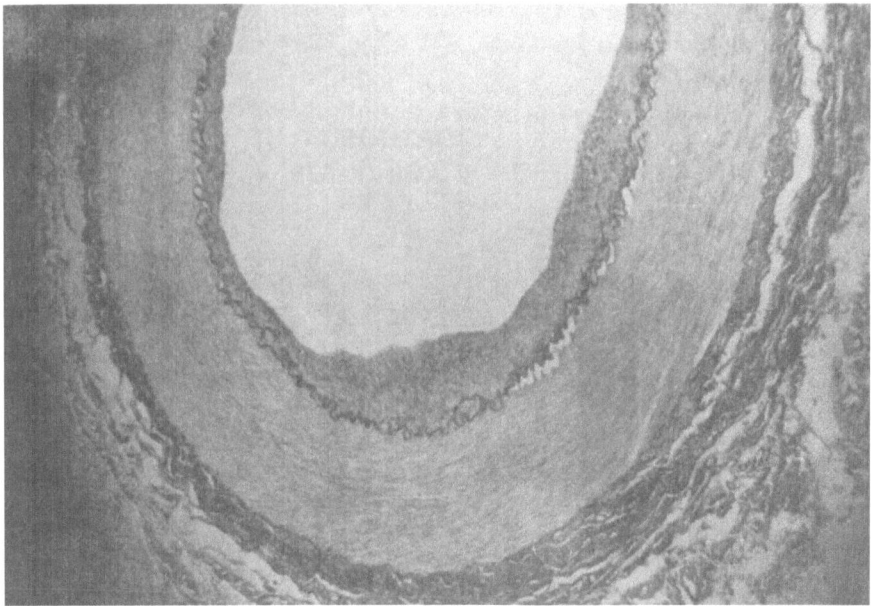

Fig. 2. Superficial temporal artery of a 64-year-old patient showing signs of severe arteriosclerosis. There is enormous thickening of the medial and the subintimal layers with simultaneous dilatation of the vessel but no calcifications

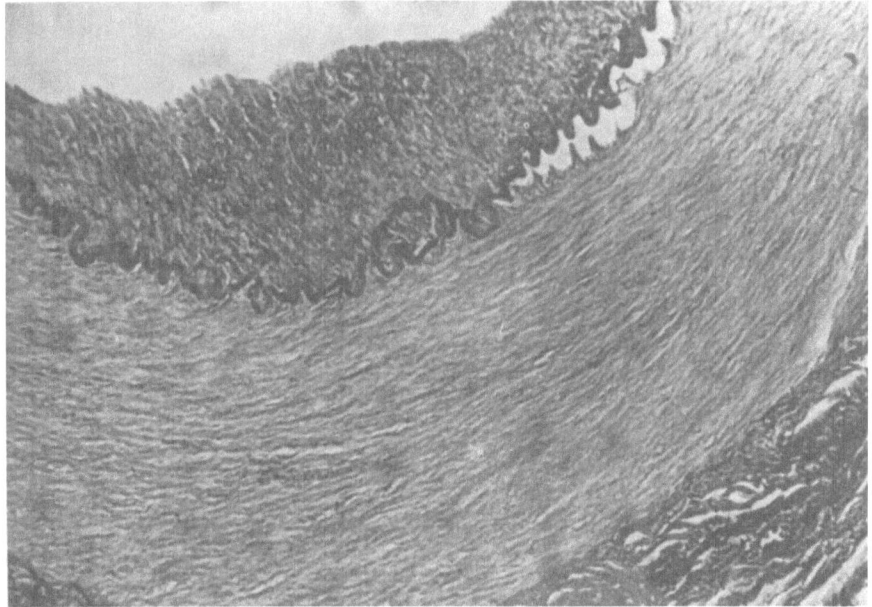

Fig. 3. Magnification of detail from Fig. 2. The elastic lamellae are clearly visible; they cause a thickening of the superficial temporal artery while allowing dilatation

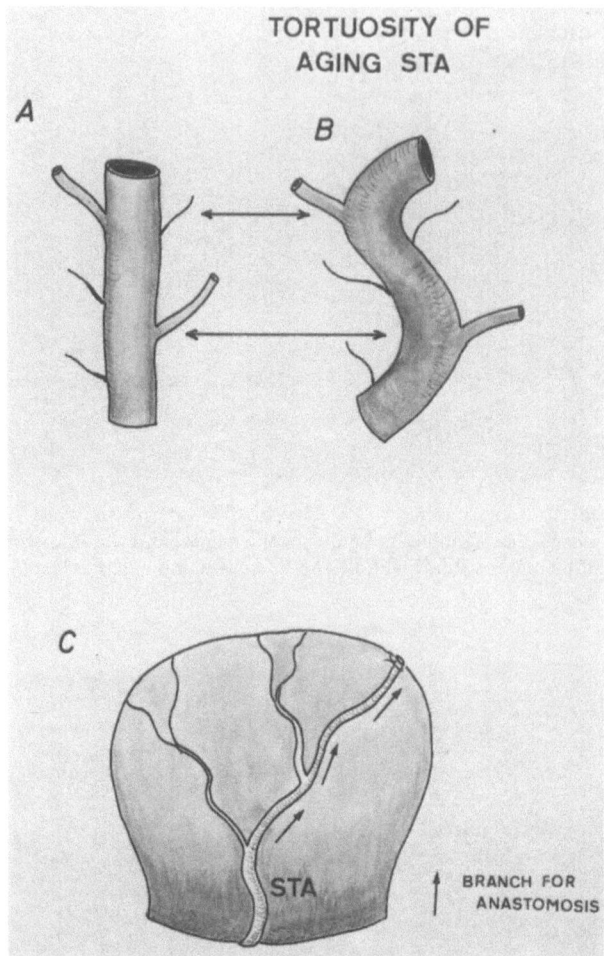

Fig. 4. Increased elastic lamellae in the superficial temporal artery and hypertension in aged patients lead to a dilatation of the vessel and to tortuosity between bifurcating branches

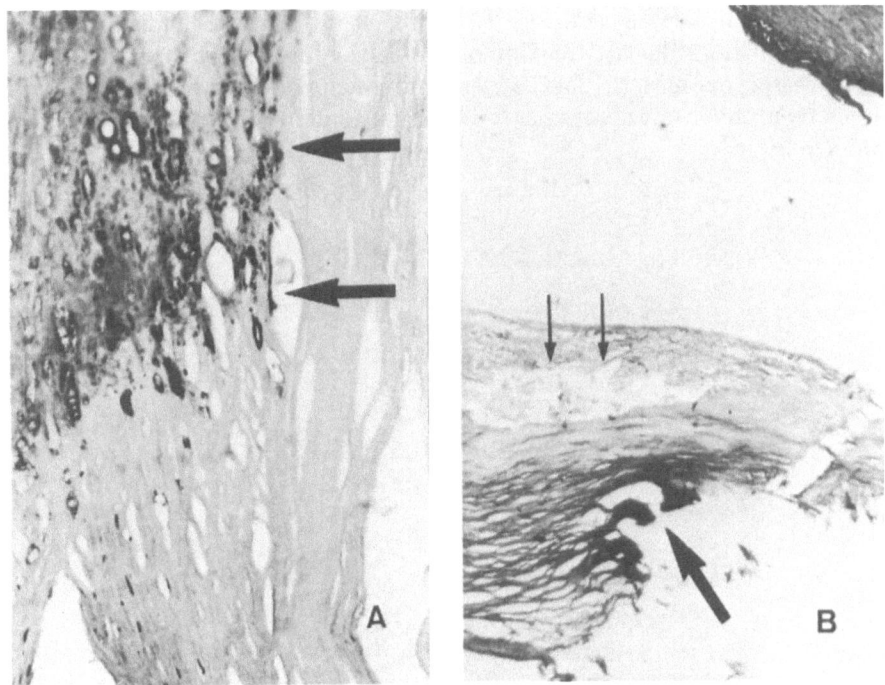

Fig. 5. Carotid bifurcation of the same patient shown in Fig. 2 and Fig. 3. Deposits of lipoid and foam cells (↑), as well as severe calcification (↑) are detectable in the wall of the carotid artery

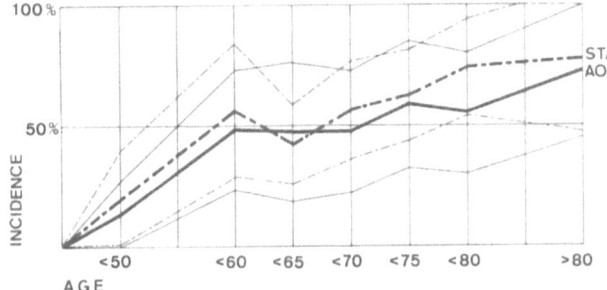

Fig. 6. The arteriosclerosis of the superficial temporal artery (*STA*) and the aorta (*AO*) is increased with the advanced age of the patient. The degree of arteriosclerosis is approximately the same in all vessels, but with varying histological changes

the form of sclerotic change. In the area of the superficial temporal artery there is an increase in elastic lamellae and a richly celled, but poorly fibered layer develops accompanied by ectasis and tortuosity of this vessel without calcifications (Fig. 4). In contrast to the superficial temporal artery, considerable calcification occurs in the internal carotid artery and other vessels examined. This causes a narrowing of the lumen which is due to sclerosis and is not compensated by enlargement of these vessels (Figs. 5 and 7).

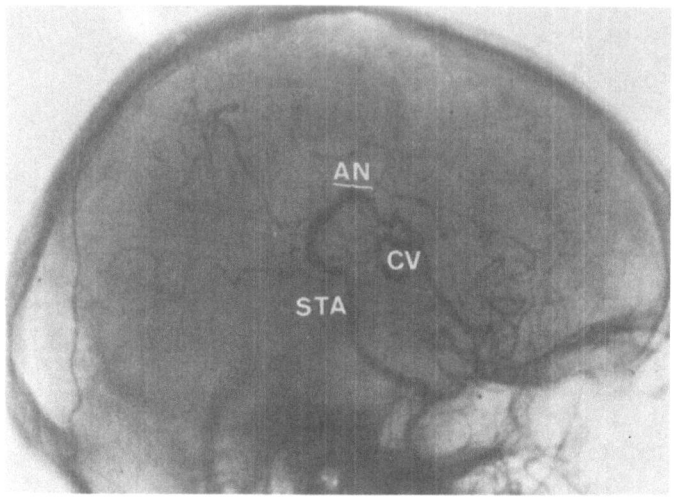

Fig. 7. Angiogram of a 56-year-old patient 12 months after extra-intracranial bypass operation for carotid occlusion. The superficial temporal artery (*STA*) has dilated enormously and is almost the size of the internal carotid artery. The cortical vessel (*CV*) is also dilated. *AN* Anastomosis

These particular pathological changes in the superficial temporal artery make this vessel very well suited for this bypass operation, especially in cases involving degenerative vascular diseases. It is of crucial importance that practically no calcification occurs; thus this vessel is able to dilate considerably in spite of slight luminal narrowing due to arteriosclerosis. If necessary, it can dilate to a diameter corresponding to that of the internal carotid artery (Fig. 7). This has been observed by all surgeons practicing extra-intracranial anastomosis. In the material under discussion, considerable luminal dilatation was also noted in all cases of extra-intracranial bypass in which the indication to operate had been correct (Kletter *et al.* 1976, 1978).

Reichmann (1975) describes a particularly pronounced dilatation of the superficial temporal artery in case 26. Yaşargil (1970) reports an enormous dilatation of the superficial temporal artery in his second operated case and stresses the importance of a satisfactory postoperative pulsation. The same view is taken by Acland (1972), Yonekawa and Yaşargil (1976), and Deruty *et al.* (1976), who also specifically mention the dilatation of the superficial temporal artery. They also indicate that this dilatation is accompanied by an extension of the supplied vascular area in the ensuing months. An excessive dilatation of the superficial temporal artery is mentioned by Chater (1972) in case 4; the lumen of the superficial temporal artery reached three times its preoperative size, as demonstrated angiographically. This author has made a similar observation (Fig. 7). This capacity to dilate requires subtile suture techniques when anastomosis is performed because *widening of the vessels is impossible* or proceeds only with difficulty *if a stenosis exists at the anastomosis site.* Therefore, if there is no or only slight dilatation of the superficial temporal artery within 4 to 6 weeks after the operation, it is due to either an incorrect indication for surgery or a faulty suture technique (Chapter 6, page 39). The importance of a special surgical technique will be discussed in detail in Chapters 6 and 8.

At the Department of Neurosurgery, Vienna, it is routine to examine histologically a small portion of the superficial temporal artery in External-Internal-Bypass-Operations. Temporal arteritis was not diagnosed in any of over 150 such examinations. In none of the publications available on extra-intracranial bypass operation is an *arteritis temporalis* reported. The cause of this affliction continues to be unknown (Gutrecht 1970, Smith and Dalessio 1972). Considering its low incidence, this pathological change of the superficial temporal artery is unlikely to be found in extra-intracranial anastomosis; however, this possibility should never be excluded. Therefore, we are in favor of submitting a small portion of the superficial temporal artery for histological examination. This also permits determination of the degree of arteriosclerosis in the patient.

4.2. The Occipital Artery

The occipital artery (Fig. 1) has its origin on the dorsal side of the external carotid artery, usually opposite the facial artery. It extends beneath the mastoideal venter of the biventer muscle in a cranial direction up to the transverse process of the atlas; it then assumes a dorsal direction. Covered by the sternocleidomastoid and the splenius muscles, it continues toward the sulcus of the occipital artery in the temporal bone. It then changes its direction at the medial edge of the splenius muscle, piercing through the trapezial muscle at its point of attachment. It courses just beneath the skin surface at the back of the head in a parietal direction, and finally splits into numerous branches.

The occipital artery's histological characteristics correspond to those of the superficial temporal artery.

In extra-intracranial anastomosis, this vessel is used only in exceptional cases, such as when the superficial temporal artery cannot be used or an alternative to an occluded anastomosis of the superficial temporal artery is needed (Spetzler 1976, Kletter 1978). The occipital artery is not very well suited for extra-intracranial anastomosis, mainly because it is partly covered by muscle tissue. For this reason, exposing it is somewhat more difficult than exposing the superficial temporal artery.

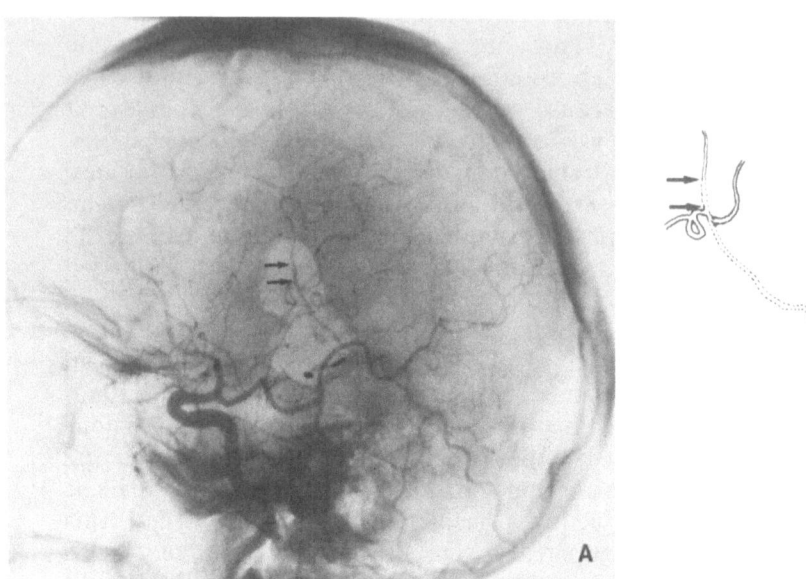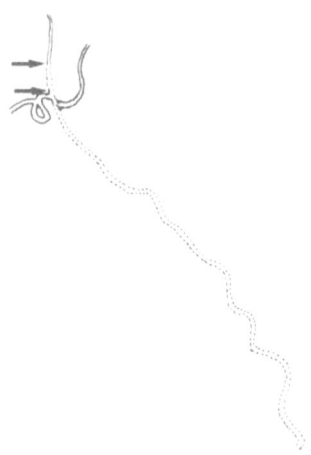

Fig. 8. Anastomosis (↑↑) between the occipital artery and a branch of the middle cerebral artery 3 weeks after operation on a 54-year-old patient with carotid occlusion. The post-operative angiogram shows only a slight dilatation of the occipital artery

Furthermore, according to the literature and this author's own experience, the dilatation capacity of the occipital artery is not as great as that of the superficial temporal artery (Spetzler 1976, Kletter 1978) (Fig. 8).

4.3. The Carotid Artery

The internal carotid artery runs from the common carotid artery, at the level of the cranial edge of the thyroid cartilage, in an almost straight course toward the external aperture of the carotid canal; it then enters the carotic canal and finally arrives at the carotid groove of the sphenoid bone, where it extends within the cavernous sinus.

Above the lacerum foramen, it ascends in an almost vertical direction, following a groove of the side surface of the body of the sphenoid; it is now adjacent to the frontal pole of the gasserian ganglion. The internal carotid artery then turns rostral and runs in a sagittal direction, slightly ascending as it extends toward the root of the anterior clinoid process. In this part of the cavernous sinus, it runs in a groove of the side wall of the body of the sphenoid on either side of the hypophyseal fossa. Below the root of the anterior clinoid process, the internal carotid artery makes a sharp turn whose convex part is directed forward (carotid knee). It is then seen below the optic nerve after penetrating the dura.

The artery then continues its course in the subarachnoidal space (cisternal part). Between the apex of the pyramid and the root of the

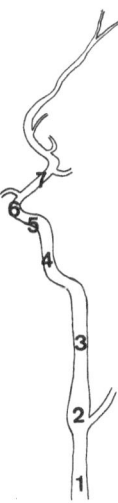

Fig. 9. Various sections of the internal carotid artery subdivided according to structural differences of the wall (Platzer 1956). *1* Common carotid artery, *2* carotid bulb, *3* internal carotid artery, extracranial part, *4* internal carotid artery in the carotid canal, *5* internal carotid artery in the cavernous sinus, *6* exit of internal carotid artery from the cavernous sinus, *7* internal carotid artery in the subarachnoid space and carotid bifurcation

anterior clinoid process, the internal carotid artery runs within the cavernous sinus, surrounded by its venous spaces and its fibrous trabecular framework.

The vessel's curviform part before, within, and above the cavernous sinus was called "carotid siphon" by Moniz. This term has since found general acceptance.

Before bifurcating into the anterior cerebral artery and the middle cerebral artery, the internal carotid artery gives off three major arteries: the ophthalmic, the posterior communicating, and the anterior choroid arteries.

Depending upon their location (extracranial, intraosseous, intracavernous, subarachnoid, or intracerebral), the vessels supplying the brain show an unusually varied structure. According to the morphology and thickness of the wall and the nature of accompanying structures, seven segments can be differentiated in the carotid artery (Fig. 9) (Platzer 1956). Within the carotid canal the adventitia and media of the internal carotid artery is gradually thinned by the loss of smooth muscle cells and collagen fibers. Although this change in the vessel wall is gradual and progressive between the entrance of the canal and the exit from the cavernous sinus, abrupt changes in structure occur at the petrous curvature and the first knee of the carotid siphon (Platzer 1957). Certainly, at the knee of the carotid siphon the loss of three-fourths of the thickness of the tunica media and tunica adventitia, the disappearance of the characteristic external limiting membrane of elastica, and the condensation of elastic fibers into the dense internal elastic layer mark the transformation of a conventional peripheral muscular artery into an intracranial artery. These changes in the wall may be due to changes in surrounding structures.

4.4. The Middle Cerebral Artery

The middle cerebral artery (Fig. 10) is the largest branch of the internal carotid, and it is the cerebral artery most often occluded. It arises lateral to the optic chiasm and passes laterally and slightly forward below the anterior perforated substance to reach the sylvian fissure. Branches arising from its superior surface penetrate the anterior perforated substance. At the base of the sylvian fissure, the middle cerebral artery begins its division into cortical arteries. While branching, the middle cerebral artery turns around the insula and courses posteriorly and superiorly in the depths of the fissure, its branches emerging to ramify over the lateral surface of the hemisphere. The middle cerebral artery may by divided into a proximal trunk and the cortical branches.

The striate arteries arise consistently from this proximal segment along its path under the anterior perforated substance. Other branches that may arise from the proximal trunk include the anterior choroid artery and a cortical branch to the tip of the temporal lobe. The choroid artery is normally considered a branch of the internal carotid but was found to arise from the middle cerebral in 11.7 percent of 60 cases studied by Carpenter et al. (1954). The artery to the temporal pole was seen to arise from the proximal trunk in one-half of the cases studied by Vander Eecken (1959) and one-fourth of those studied by Herman et al. (1963).

On reaching the sylvian fissure, the middle cerebral artery gives off its cortical branches. These supply nearly all the lateral surface of the hemisphere and the underlying white matter. The territory was accurately outlined anatomically by Beevor (1907).

The middle cerebral artery also supplies the entire insula, the lateral orbital surface of the frontal lobe, and the tip of the temporal lobe. In the last region it meets branches of the posterior cerebral and anterior choroid arteries.

Although the pattern of branching of the surface vessels is highly variable, the following arteries are reasonably constant: the temporal

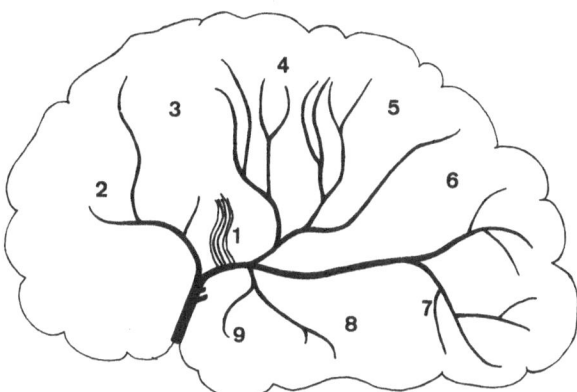

Fig. 10. Middle cerebral artery. *1* Striate arteries (perforante arteries, thalamostriate arteries, thalamolenticulare arteries, lenticulostriate arteries), *2* orbitofrontale artery (frontobasal lateral artery), *3* praecentral artery, *4* central artery, *5* parietal arteries, *6* angular artery, *7* posterior temporal artery, *8* middle temporal artery, *9* temporal polar artery. One of *the four main variations* in the pattern of the major branches of the middle cerebral artery is shown. The main temporal branch located posterior to the origin of the striate arteries

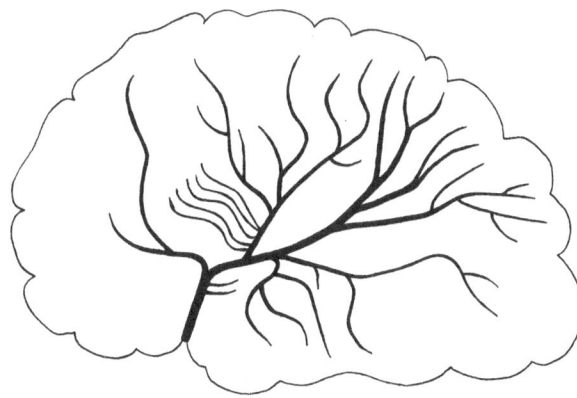

Fig. 11. *One of four main variations* in the pattern of the major branches of the middle cerebral artery: The main bifurcation is located anterior to the origin of the striate arteries

polar, anterior temporal, orbitofrontal, precentral, central, anterior parietal, posterior temporal, posterior parietal, and angular artery. Vander Eecken (1959) studied the origin and area of supply of all the cortical arteries in 40 cases while examining the anastomoses between these vessels.

The temporal polar artery, an inconstant branch found in 22 of 40 cases by Vander Eecken (1959), is seen to arise from the proximal trunk

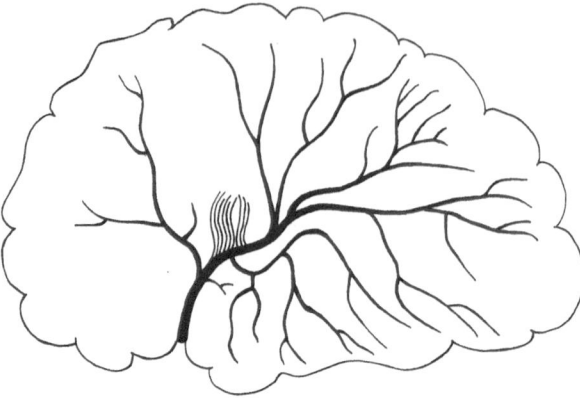

Fig. 12. *One of four main variations* in the pattern of the major branches of the middle cerebral artery. The main temporal branch is located at the origin of the striate arteries

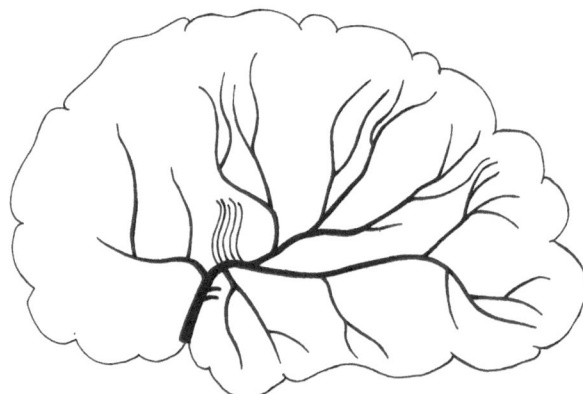

Fig. 13. *One of four main variations* in the pattern of the major branches of the middle cerebral artery. The main temporal branch is located posterior to the origin of the striate arteries; a further branch divides into the polar temporal artery and the anterior temporal artery

opposite the origin of the lateral striate arteries. It supplies the anterior tip of the temporal lobe. The anterior temporal artery is usually the next to arise. It usually supplies the anterior half of the temporal lobe. When the temporal polar artery is absent, however, the anterior temporal supplies the temporal pole as well.

The middle cerebral artery has its first main bifurcation at the base of the insula. This division forms two groups of arteries: the anterior and the posterior. The anterior group includes the orbitofrontal, precentral, central, and anterior parietal arteries.

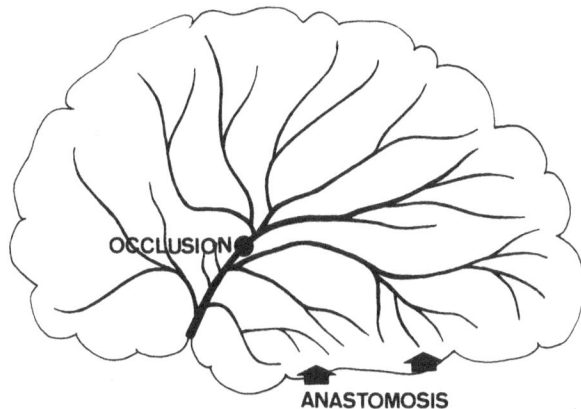

OCCLUSION

ANASTOMOSIS

Fig. 14. In the event of a distal occlusion of the middle cerebral artery and proximal bifurcation of the temporal branches, an anastomosis with the cortical branches of the profound temporal artery is useless. This anastomosis would not be capable of supplying the region of the angular artery

After the branching off of the ascending trunk, the middle cerebral artery usually runs into the depths of the lateral fissure and forms the branches of the posterior group: the posterior parietal, posterior temporal, parieto-occipital and angular arteries. These supply the posterior parts of the parietal and temporal lobes, parts of the lateral surface of the occipital lobe, and the posterior half of the insula.

For extra-intracranial bypass operations the vessels selected are usually in the temporal lobe or in the region of the angular artery. This is the reason that variations in the main branches of the middle cerebral artery are very important in this operation.

In 60 postmortem brains investigated by the author the variations occurred where the main temporal branch comes off the middle cerebral artery. In 32 of the 60 vessels examined, this division was located posterior to the origin of the striate arteries (Fig. 10). In 12 cases it was located anterior to the origin of the striate arteries (Fig. 11), and in 12 cases it was at the vessels themselves (Fig. 12). In 4 cases it was located posterior to the origin of the striate arteries, but there was a further branch originating in the area of these vessels and dividing into the temporal polar artery and the anterior temporal artery (Fig. 13) (Kletter 1975). If the main temporal branch is located anterior to the origin of the striate arteries and if the occlusion of the middle cerebral artery is after the bifurcation, anastomosis with a temporal artery cannot irrigate the area of the angular artery (Fig. 14). These findings show the importance of establishing the location of the arterial occlusion before selecting the vessels to be anastomosed. The correlation between the vascular lesion and the vascular anatomy is important to ensure the proper functioning of the anastomosis and to ensure irrigation of the necessary area.

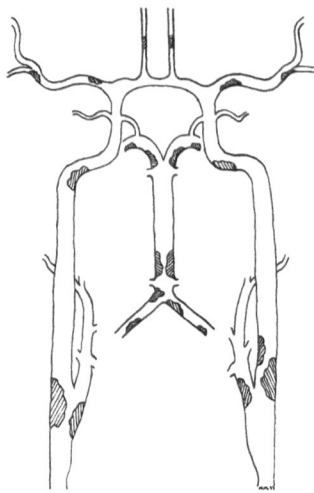

Fig. 15. Most common sites of arteriosclerosis in the carotid and vertebral regions

4.5. Physiological Arterial Anastomoses and Collateral Circulation

The four large brain vessels are connected to each other by numerous collaterals and anastomoses (Fig. 16). Thus, under certain conditions, the occlusion of a vessel can be compensated by collaterals. There are four types of anastomosis: extracranial, extra-intracranial, intracranial, and intracerebral.

Most frequently, a physiological extra-intracranial anastomosis can be observed in occlusions of the internal carotid artery. This collateral extends from the external carotid artery via the ophthalmic artery to the intracranial section of the internal carotid artery (Fig. 16/3). The blood flow to the ophthalmic artery is ensured either by the facial and angular arteries, via the superficial temporal and the supraorbital arteries, or by the maxillary artery and the middle meningeal artery. The most important intracranial anastomoses are found in the circle of Willis, particularly the anterior communicating artery (Fig. 16/1) and the posterior cerebral arteries (Fig. 16/2).

In addition to these physiological anastomoses in the basis, there are a number of meningeal anastomoses throughout the convexity of the cerebrum and the cerebellum. The three large arteries of the cerebellum form a rich network of anastomoses (Fig. 16/6) (Tschabitscher et al. 1975). Above the convexity of the cerebrum, there are many anastomoses between the anterior, middle, and posterior arteries, as well as throughout the choroid artery (Fig. 16/4).

Intracranial anastomoses are undoubtedly of greater importance from a functional point of view than those between the external carotid artery and the intracranial vessels. Whether these collaterals are hemodynamically sufficient depends greatly on the time factor and the original size of the anastomoses. The anatomical presence of collaterals does not necessarily prove their actual ability to function. In general, there is a correlation between the size and capacity of angiographic anastomoses

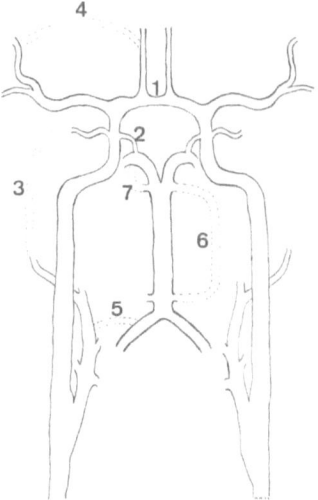

Fig. 16. The most important collaterals in cases of stenoses and occlusions of the cerebral arteries in the order of their importance: *1* anterior communicating artery, *2* posterior communicating artery, *3* ophthalmic artery, *4* cortical anastomoses between the area of the anterior cerebral artery and the middle cerebral artery region, *5* anastomoses between the vertebral artery and the external carotid artery, *6* cortical anastomoses in the region of the cerebellar arteries, *7* anastomoses between the occipital lobe and cerebellar arteries

and the degree of clinical disturbances (Tönnis and Schiefer 1959, Krayenbühl and Yaşargil 1963). If a vascular occlusion progresses gradually, there is sufficient time for a collateral circulation to develop, if such collaterals exist. If the vascular change sets in suddenly, it is very difficult for collaterals to replace the previous circulation. If systemic blood pressure has decreased because of these changes the resistance of the peripheral vessels cannot be sufficiently overcome.

Thus, in the case of a cerebrovascular occlusion, various factors determine whether a functional or a structural deficit will occur: the patient's age and general condition, his blood pressure, the condition of the arteries, the type of occlusion and its location, the number of existing collaterals, and the reactivity and regulatory capacity of the affected cerebral parenchyma.

5. Experimental Surgery

The end-to-end anastomosis of vessels with a diameter of 1 mm or less is an extremely difficult technique (Jacobson *et al.* 1960; 1962; Yaşargil 1967; Piza-Katzer 1974). It requires thorough training. The common carotid artery of the rat is best suited for this purpose. In regard to its size and consistency, this vessel is comparable to those used in extra-intracranial anastomosis. Moreover, the changes caused by aging and by chronic hypertension produce morphological changes similar to those that take place in human vessels of the same diameter (Meyermann and Kletter 1977; Meyermann *et al.* 1977). Another advantage is that rats present no particular difficulties either as test animals or during the operation in comparison with other small experimental animals such as hares and cats. End-to-end microvascular anastomoses are performed on the arteries of hares, ears, however, mainly to practice plastic and reconstructive surgery (Buncke and Schultz 1965).

5.1. Microvascular Anastomoses on the Common Carotid Artery of the Rat

5.1.1. End-to-End Anastomosis

After narcosis by intraperitoneal administration of an anesthetic, the animal is affixed to a plate of glass or wood by immobilization of its extremities. A transverse skin incision is then made from one shoulder joint to the other. It is advisable to strip up a broad portion of the skin in both directions, in order to obtain a good view of the cervical muscles (Fig. 18). After the superficial cervical fascia is exposed, the incision is prolonged between the sterno-cleidomastoid muscle and the cervical muscles (Fig. 19). This procedure is performed under the operating microscope. A transverse muscle invariably found above the common carotid artery can be severed without damage to the test animal.

The common carotid artery is accompanied by a relatively thick vagus nerve (Fig. 20). This can be used as an indication of direction. The common carotid artery should be dissected from the surrounding connective tissue as much as possible. Occasionally, the bifurcation of this artery, into its two branches is located at a greater depth, so that certain difficulties may arise in exposing it. It is advisable to place a small piece of glove rubber cut in a triangular shape under the artery, after complete exposure of this vessel, in order to protect the surrounding tissue. This measure also helps to locate small fibrous adhesions to the posterior wall of the vessel or

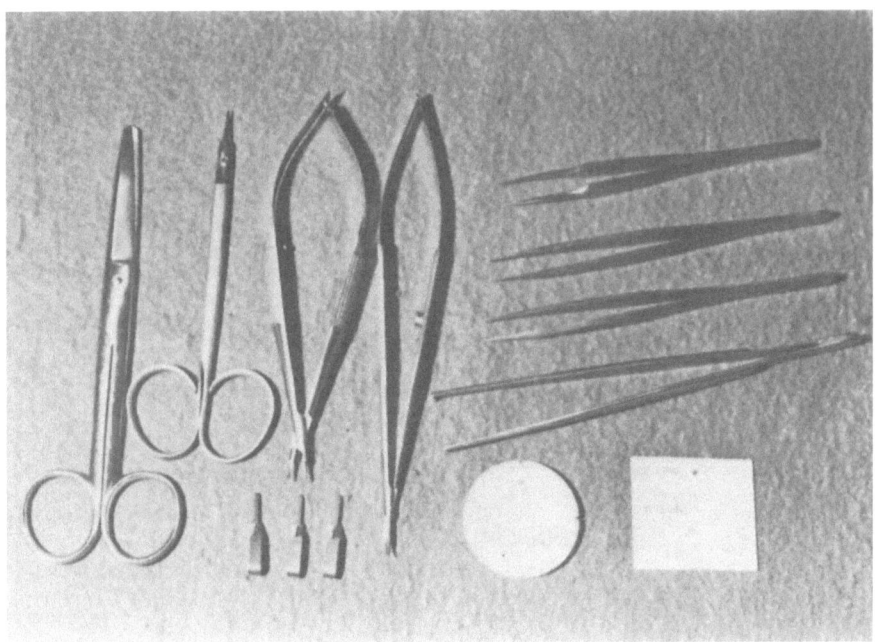

Fig. 17. Instruments for microanastomoses on the carotid artery of the rat

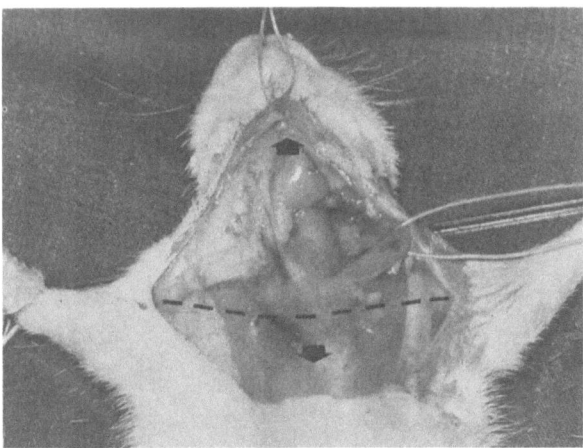

Fig. 18. Immobilization of the test animal and skin incision for the exposure of the common carotid artery. Cranial and caudal stripping of the skin for exposure of the cervical muscles

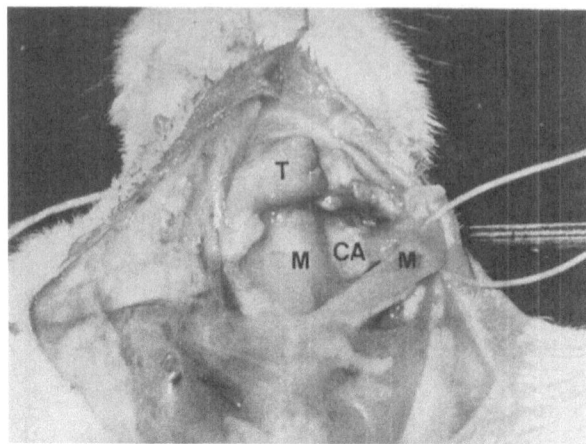

Fig. 19. Access to the common carotid artery (*CA*) of the rat between the cervical
muscles (*M*). (*T* salivary gland)

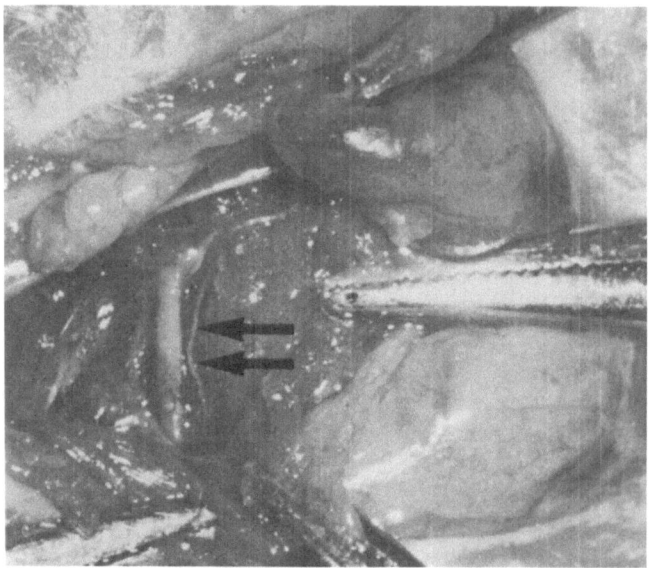

Fig. 20. Exposed common carotid artery of the rat with vagus nerve (↑↑)

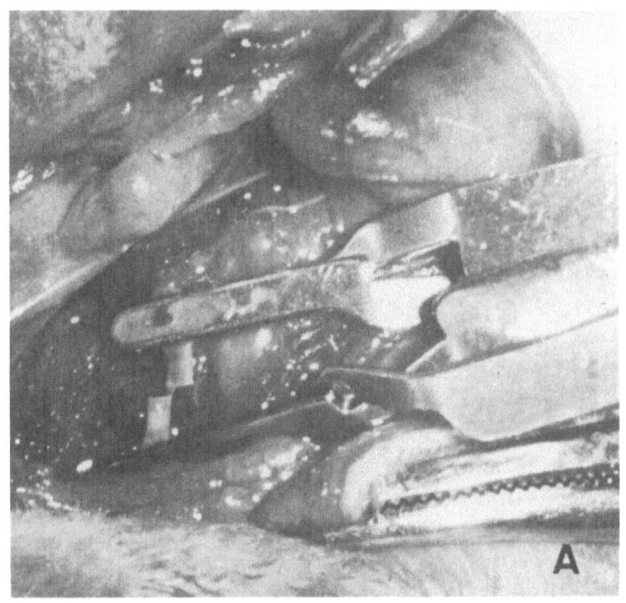

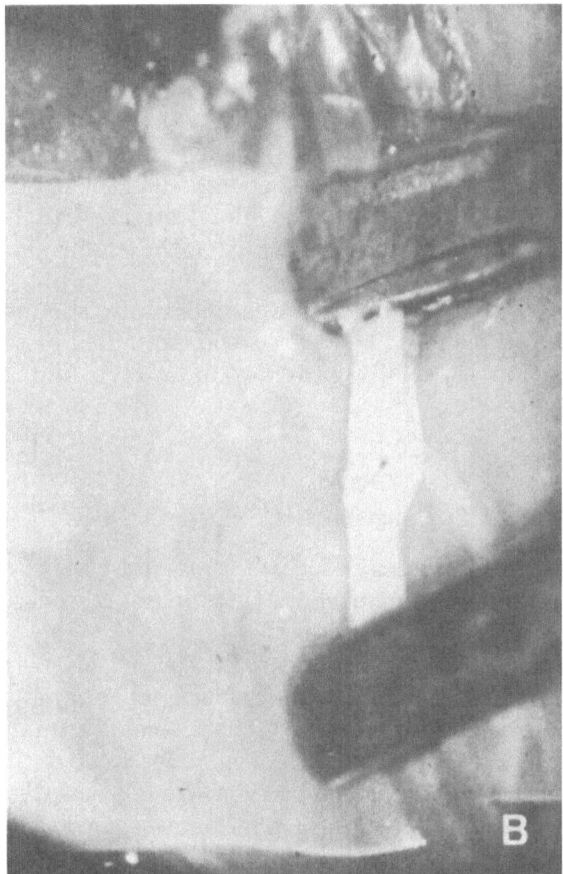

Fig. 21. After application of the corner sutures, first the anterior and then the posterior
wall is sutured

small vascular bifurcations, which then require appropriate action. The vessel is then clamped, severed, and connected with 10-0 suture material. The classical technique (Jacobson and Suarez 1960, Buncke and Schultz 1965, Acland 1972) consists of first applying two corner sutures at an angle of 180 degrees and then suturing the anterior and the posterior walls (Fig. 21 B).

5.1.2. End-to-Side Anastomosis

For extra-intracranial anastomosis operation it is advisable to practice end-to-side anastomosis. A technique introduced by this author on the carotid artery of the rat allows a successful end-to-side anastomosis with satisfactory postoperative functioning. The suturing technique in this operation is similar to that used in end-to-end anastomosis.

The common carotid arteries are exposed bilaterally as described above. The common carotid artery of one side is ligated distally and proximally and then extirpated and placed into a physiological saline solution.

The common carotid artery of the opposite side is clamped proximally and distally, and a longitudinal incision is made at two points (Fig. 22). The contralateral common carotid artery is now implanted as a flat loop onto the clamped vessel (Fig. 23). This requires two end-to-side anastomoses. The clamped vessel is then ligated in the middle. If both end-to-side anastomoses are patent, the blood stream can be clearly seen flowing through the artificial bypass after the clamp has been opened (Fig. 24).

About 1 week after the operation, angiography should be performed and the anastomoses should be excised and examined histologically. The latter examination especially provides data revealing an inadequate suture technique.

5.2. Experimental Studies in Dogs

The experimental studies described above may serve as preliminary tests but are of limited value because they do not completely correspond to physiological conditions in humans.

In order to ascertain whether end-to-end or end-to-side anastomosis is preferable, anastomosis between the superficial temporal artery and a large branch of the middle cerebral artery or its main trunk was performed by several authors (Yaşargil and Denton 1974; Kletter und Koos 1975) (Fig. 25). Anastomoses performed on dogs are not suitable as models for the treatment of cerebral infarction in humans because the cerebral blood supply in dogs is different. Nonetheless, this experimental test is very useful for perfecting and studying the surgical technique. This method presents considerable technical difficulties, however, because the vessels

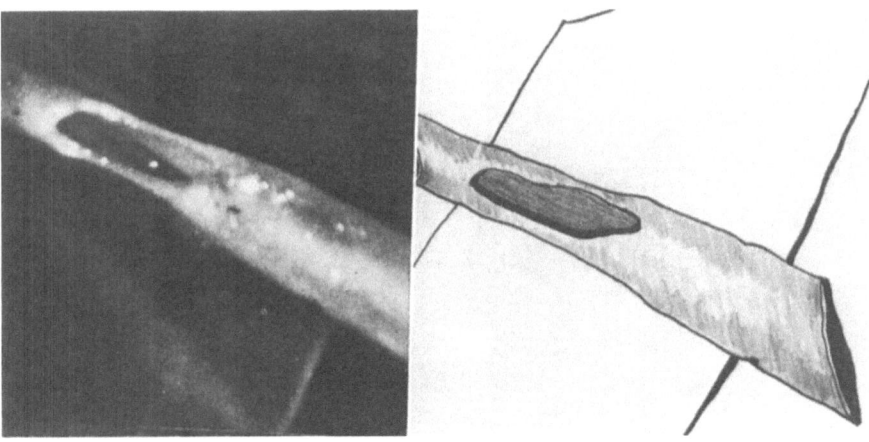

Fig. 22. Incision of the common carotid artery of the rat

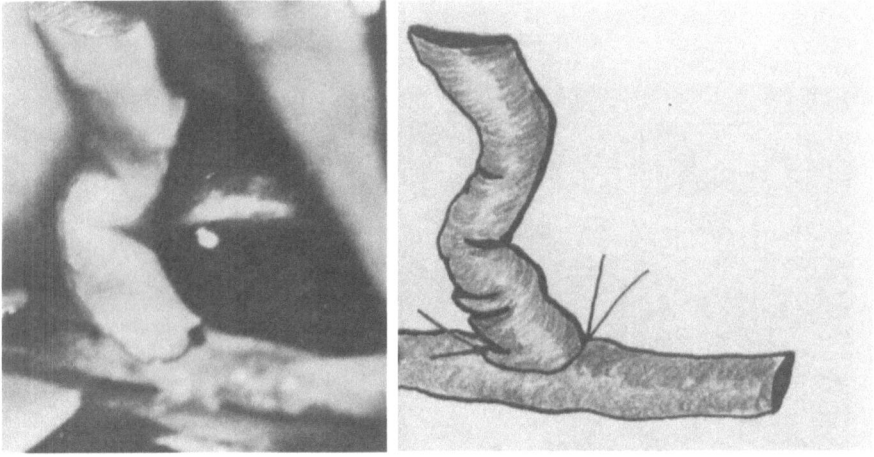

Fig. 23. Transplantation of the contralateral common carotid artery onto the exposed and clamped common carotid artery by means of two end-to-side anastomoses

involved have a diameter of about 0.5 mm. The purpose of this investigation was also to determine the effects of superficial temporal artery-cortical microanastomoses on cerebral blood flow and its autoregulation (Fein and Molinari 1976). After experimental occlusion of the middle cerebral artery and its subsequent reopening a luxury perfusion syndrome (Lassen *et al.* 1963) was observed.

The increase in blood flow observed in the post-temporal-cortical anastomosis was relatively and absolutely greater and at higher pCO_2 values than those in the control studies (Fein and Molinari 1976).

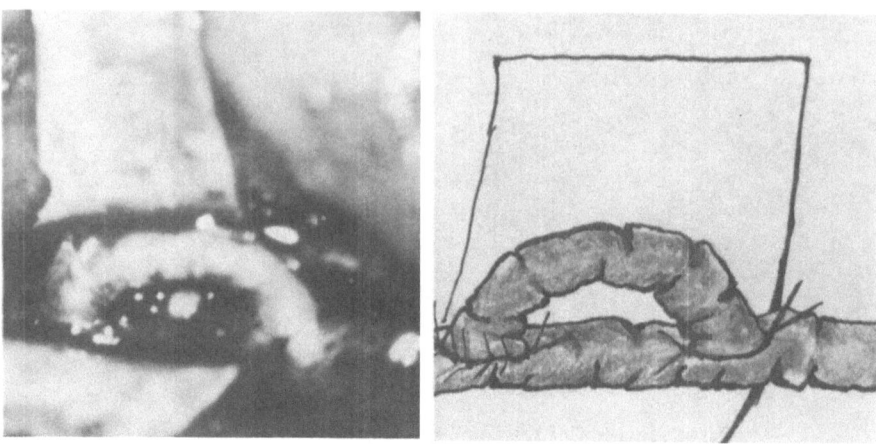

Fig. 24. After opening the clamps a good filling of the transplanted vessel is visible

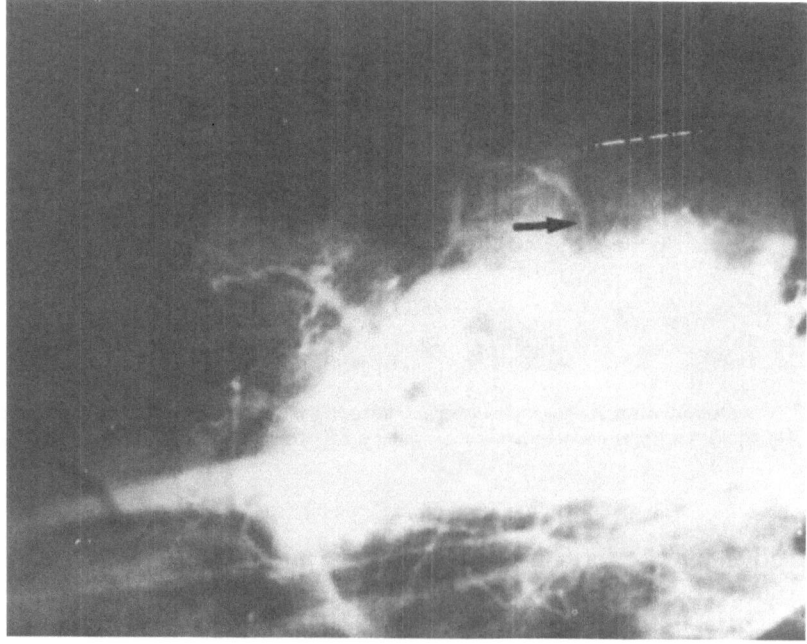

Fig. 25. Anastomosis (↑) between the temporal artery and a branch of the middle cerebral
artery of a dog

5.3. Conclusion

Experimental surgery on dogs is not required training for extra-intracranial anastomosis, although it may be used for preliminary studies such as cerebral blood flow and its autoregulation. The temporal-cortical anastomosis in dogs is a difficult technique and is good training for this type of operation.

It is absolutely essential to practice end-to-end and end-to-side microvascular anastomoses on rats in order to develop an accurate surgical technique and to learn how to handle the operating microscope. The surgeon's own technique may be further refined by conducting postoperative evaluations, such as fluorescein angiography, angiography or histological examinations, and then correlating the results with the suture technique. This will greatly reduce the likelihood of postoperative shunt deficiencies.

6. Pathophysiology of Microanastomoses

6.1. Histological Changes in Microvascular Anastomoses

Histological studies of microvascular anastomoses have been conducted by only a few authors (Baxter *et al.* 1972; Bannister 1974, 1976, 1977; Kletter and Meyermann 1974, 1976, 1977; Meyermann and Kletter 1975, 1977). More than 500 sutured end-to-end and end-to-side anastomoses on the carotid artery of the rat were performed by the author and Dr. Meyermann, Department of Neuropathology, University of Göttingen Medical School. The functional performance varied between a minimum of less than 1 hour and a maximum of 22 months (observed in two animals).

After *24 hours*, degeneration and desintegration processes were predominant at the sites of the microanastomoses. Each lesion of vascular wall was covered by a thrombus. This stage lasted approximately 3 days (Figs. 26, 28).

After *36 hours*, connective tissue cells appeared increasingly at the marginal zone of the necrosis or the incipient necrosis. After 48 hours, new endothelium began to develop. This process was partially completed at the end of the first week (Fig. 28).

After *5 to 7 days*, a total necrosis, characterized by a disappearance of all structures of the evaginated vascular walls, was observed. The connective tissue was proliferating massively, and the necrosis began organizing.

The necroses that developed in the area of the sutures were terminated after 1 week. At this time, some connective tissue had spread out from the margin, so that a dehiscence was prevented, at least, we did not observe any dehiscence at a later period.

After *7 to 14 days*, the organization reached its climax with the formation of foreignbody giant cells around the suture material (Fig. 29). At this stage, the thrombi were considerably retracted and covered with a new intima.

After approximately *14 days*, a bridge of connective tissue, which at first stretched to far beyond the periadventitia, was clearly visible between the vessel ends. This fibrous bridge clearly diminished in size during the first 2 to 3 months (Fig. 30). Even *after 4 to 6 months* it was still evident and was not incorporated into the normal vascular wall. The assumption that such a massive fibrous reaction at the site of the anastomosis could later cause a narrowing of the lumen, due to shrinkage of the connective tissue, was not confirmed. In our opinion, it was due to permanent pressure on the vascular wall coming from the inside. This

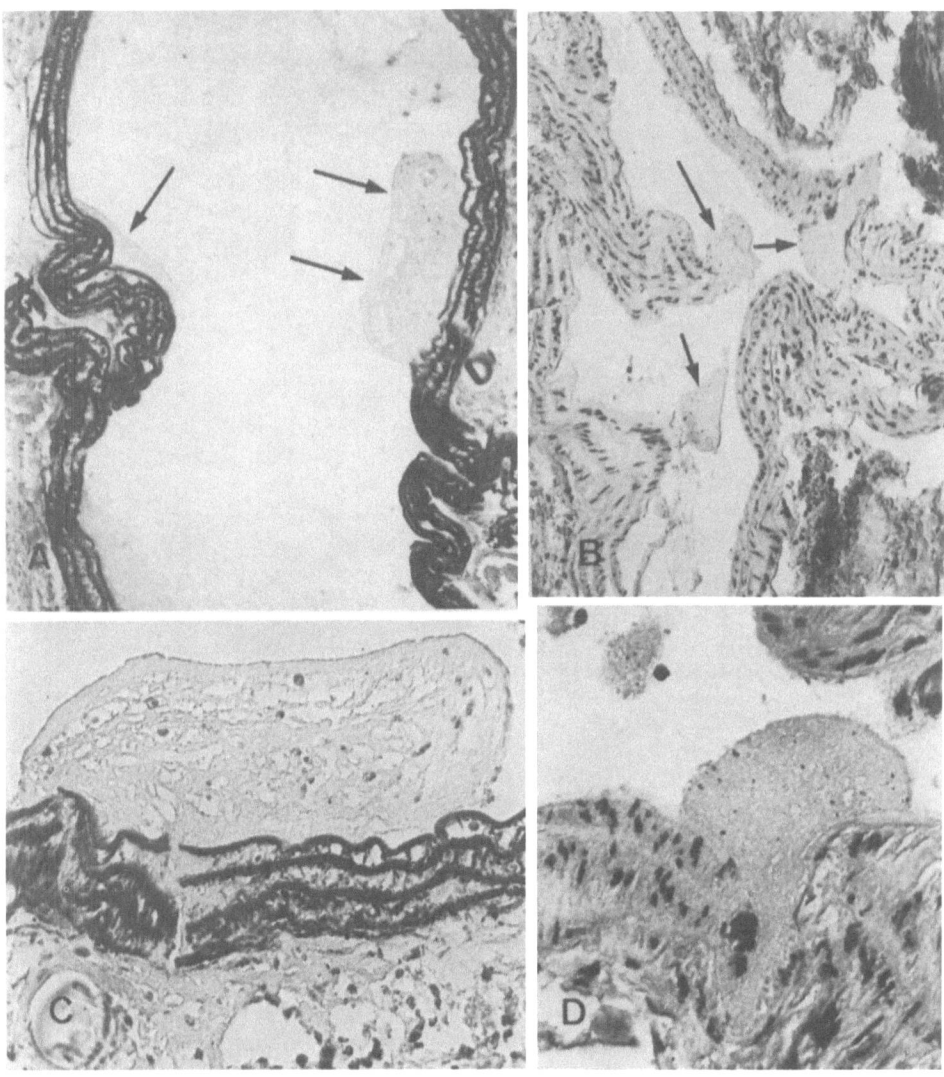

Fig. 26. Formation of thrombi above mural lesions

pressure prevented an excessive shrinkage of the connective tissue during the primary stage of regeneration in the first months. Our electron microscopic examinations revealed considerable widening of the subendothelial space. This change is usually noted only in very old vessels and has to be considered a direct consequence of microvascular anastomosis. Furthermore, a proliferation of specific organelles was observed (Meyermann and Kletter 1976; Meyermann et al. 1978).

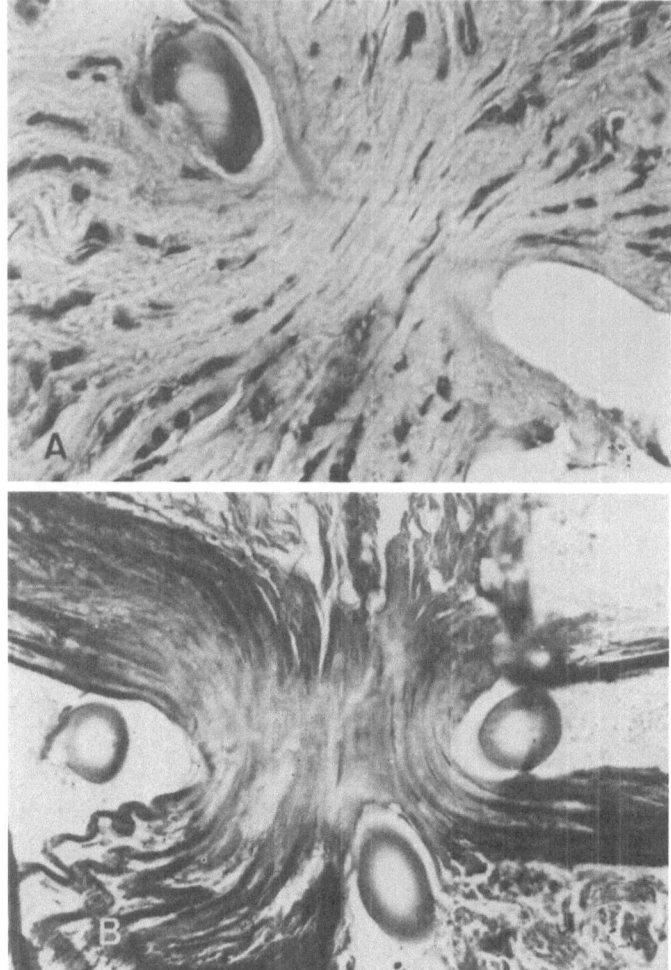

Fig. 27. Formation of necroses at the sutures 48 hours (A) and 72 hours (B) after microanastomosis, H. E. × 80

These studies had never before, to the author's knowledge, been carried out over such a long period of time. They demonstrated that a continuous disintegration and a regeneration of lesioned tissue structures occurred after an anastomosis on microvessels. In the area of the suture, a total necrosis took place within the first 24 to 48 hours. This must be considered a result of pressure exerted by the surgical knots. This pressure necrosis could not be prevented by alterating the suture technique. During the first few postoperative hours, each lesion was covered by a small or larger thrombus (Fig. 26). These thrombi were particularly large whenever histological examination showed a slight dehiscence of the wall.

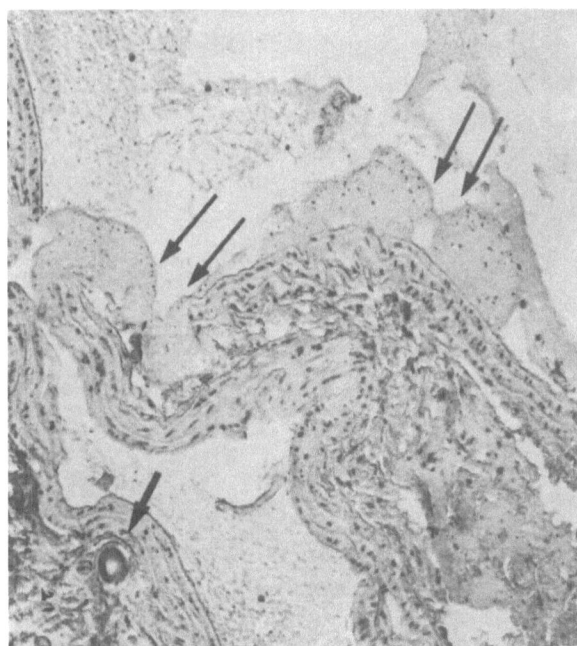

Fig. 28. Incipient organization of existing microthrombi accompanied by incipient re-endothelialization. H. E. × 60

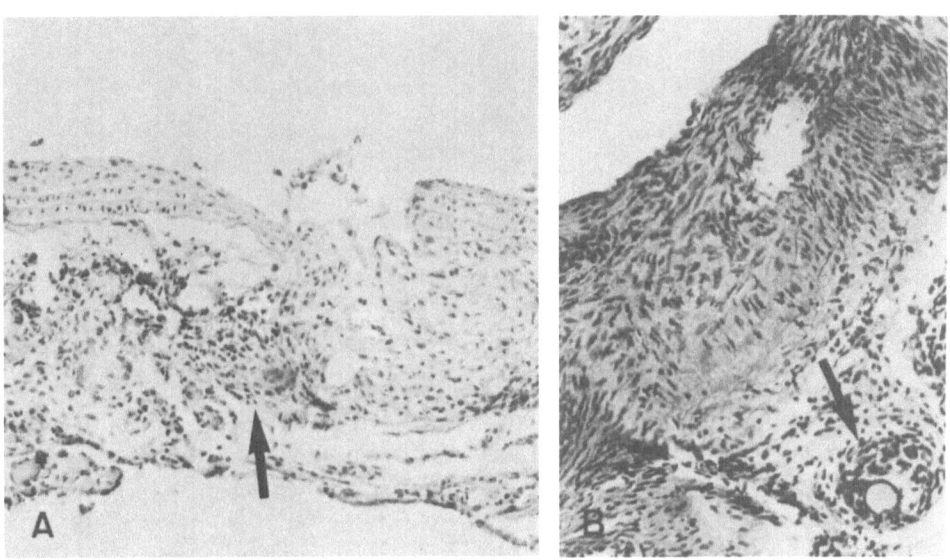

Fig. 29. Microanastomosis after 14 days. Massive fibrous proliferation is seen at the anastomosis site, double the size of the vascular wall. Formation of foreign body giant cells has occurred around the suture material (↑). H. E. × 80

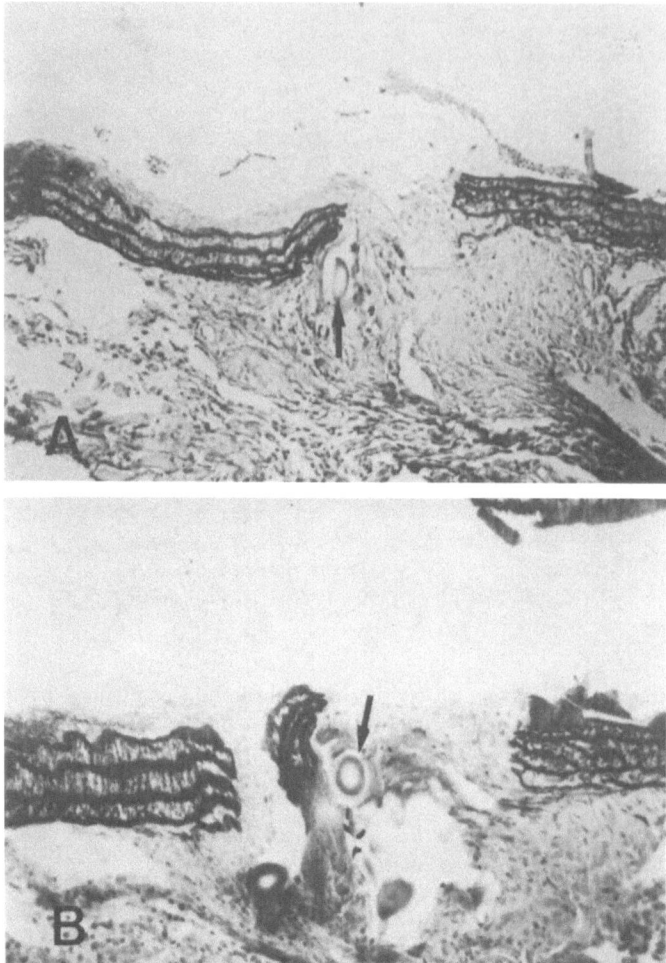

Fig. 30. A) Microanastomosis after 3 months. A large fibrous band connects the vessel ends. Suture material is seen in the connective tissue (↑). The whole lesion is covered with intima; the vascular lumen is not narrowed. B) Anastomosis after 5 months. Changes correspond to those in panel A. van Gieson × 60

We correlated these experimental and histological results with a histological examination of 4 patients who died several months after microvascular anastomosis surgery. The histological findings were approximately the same as those of a comparable experimental period.

6.2. Causes of Stenoses and Occlusions in Microsurgical Anastomoses

Histological examinations have shown that the most important stages of repair and regeneration take place in the first 48 hours, and then in the following 5 days. To a decisive degree, stenoses and occlusions at the sites of anastomoses occur during this period of time. A dilatation and readjustment of the lumen is distinctly visible after an initial narrowing during the first 48 hours. This was also observed clinically following the extra-intracranial bypass operation.

Suture dehiscences proved to be the most frequent cause of disfunction. They caused hemorrhaging into the surrounding area. If the bleeding persisted and was not contained surgically, it developed into a

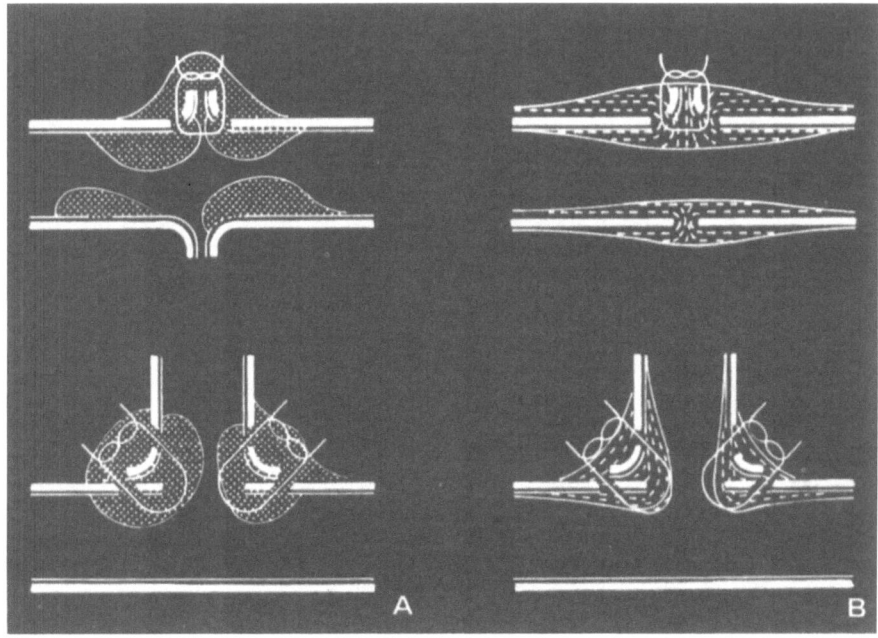

Fig. 31. A) Preferred location of new thrombi in end-to-end (upper part) and end-to-side anastomoses (lower part). B) The thrombi retract within 14 days and are organized by connective tissue. At this stage, the changes correspond histologically to those in Figs. 29 and 30

thrombus at the outer wall of the vessel. A dehiscent vascular wall may cause the thrombus to project into the interior of the vessel and cause primary occlusion of that vessel (Fig. 32). In any case, the suture dehiscence caused a considerable primary stenosis at the site of anastomosis. Oversuturing of the bleeding dehiscent area very often leads to stenosis, since there is practically no visibility at this site due to the bleeding. Part of the vascular wall may then invaginate or excess suture material may enter into the lumen. On the other hand, if the vascular section is clamped, the short stasis of the blood stream very often causes a primary thrombosis or increases thrombophilia around the small mural lesions.

Invagination of the vascular wall and temporary clamping of the vessel section in question was also thrombogenetic (Fig. 33).

Mural lesions, caused by careless handling of forceps or clamps, ranked as the second most common cause of microanastomotic failure. Frequently, a small thrombus was observed above the small lesions brought about by the suture material (Fig. 26 A, C).

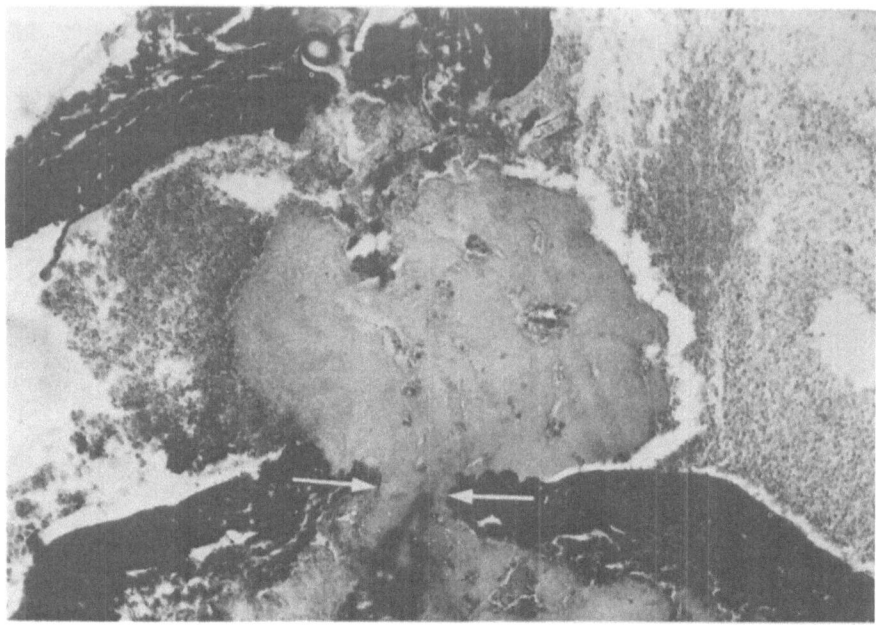

Fig. 32. Massive thrombus formation and almost complete occlusion of the microanastomosis due to suture dehiscence. The suture dehiscence (↑↑) has caused bleeding and thus thrombus formation inside and outside the vessel. H. E. × 60

Another factor leading to inadequate function was intrusion of *foreign matter into the lumen*. An invaginated vascular wall must also be regarded as foreign matter, because even when they projected only slightly into the lumen, vascular walls caused severe thrombotic changes (Fig. 33). When too much suture material was used, thrombotic changes occurred around these sutures. These sutures also have to be considered as foreign matter (Fig. 34).

Inadequately sutured anastomoses also produced a massive perivascular fibrous mantle, which under certain hemodynamic conditions caused stenosis of the anstomosis at the suture site.

The present results showed that the functional performance of a microvascular anastomosis is dependent mainly on accurate suture

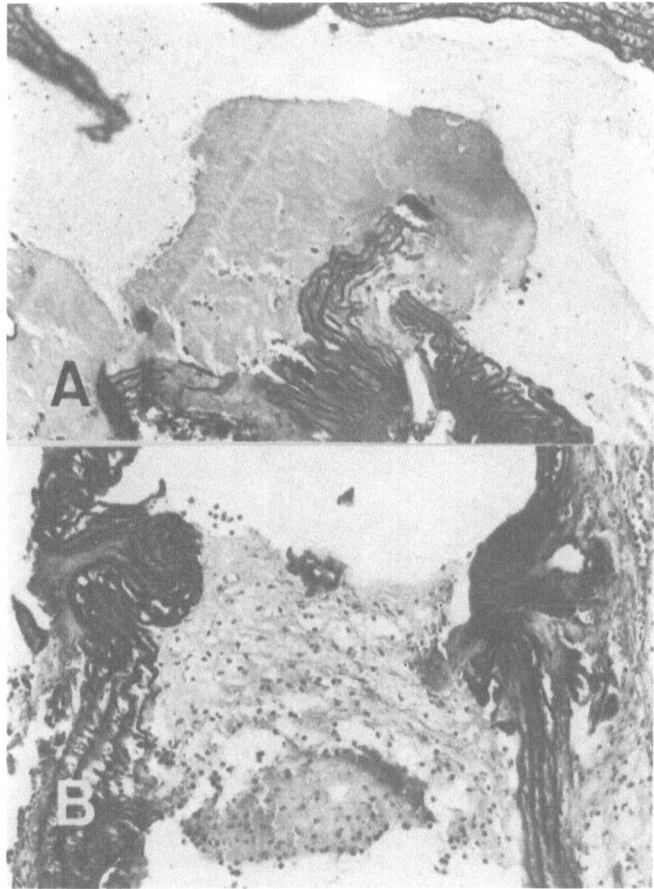

Fig. 33. A) Thrombus formation near the invaginated vascular wall. B) Medium-sized flow obstacles can also cause a complete occlusion of the microanastomosis. Elastica × 80

technique. Failures were due to thrombotic changes occurring during the first few days following small vessel anastomosis. If only stenosis and no occlusion took place, then later changes consisted of a massive formation of new fibrous tissue. In the event of poor hemodynamic function, stenosis or occlusion of the anastomosis may occur at a later date. From the present study it may be concluded that the expertise of the surgeon has a particular influence on the microanastomotic function.

The most frequent causes of microanastomotic failure due to surgery may be summarized as follows:

1. Suture dehiscence.
2. Mural lesions (outside the anastomosis).
3. Foreign matter (invaginated vascular wall, excess suture material).

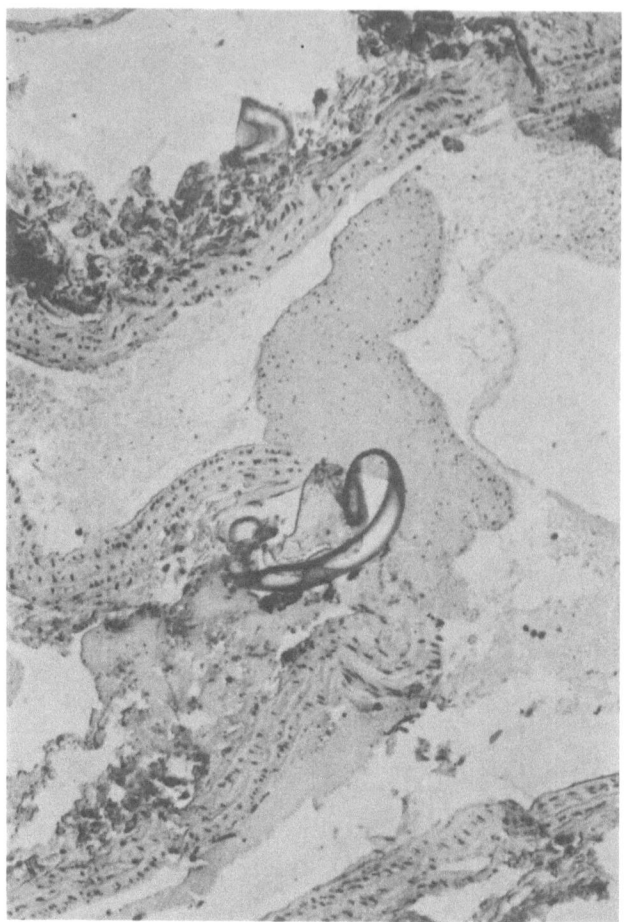

Fig. 34. End-to-side anastomosis. Considerable thrombus formation has been caused by large amounts of suture material (secondary suture applied after occurrence of suture dehiscence and bleeding from the anastomosis). The microanastomosis has been almost completely occluded by a thrombus. H. E. × 60

6.3. Relationship Between Suturing Technique, Pathohistology, and Blood Flow

Stenosis at the site of anastomosis can be brought about by:

1. an excessively narrow end-to-side anastomosis,

2. histological changes caused by severe mural trauma accompanied by considerable formation of thrombi in the area of the anastomosis, or

3. late changes due to heavy fibrous proliferation (excess foreign matter or local infection).

The superficial temporal artery has a remarkable dilating capacity of up to four times its lumen (Chapter 4.1., page 12). This fact must be taken into consideration when an extra-intracranial anastomosis is performed. The same is true for the cortical artery. If a stenosis exists at the site of anastomosis, however, these vessels will be unable to dilate. For this reason, an essential precondition for subsequent full functioning of the

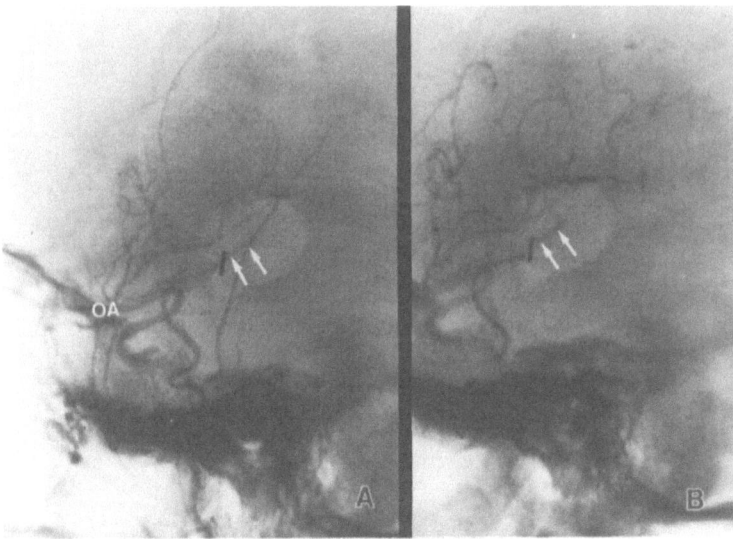

Fig. 35. Carotid angiogram 4 weeks after extra-intracranial anastomosis in a 56-year-old patient with carotid occlusion on the left and satisfactory collateral circulation via the ophthalmic artery. A) In the initial stage there was good supply of the carotid siphon and the initial part of the middle cerebral artery, as well as irrigation of the superficial temporal artery up to the anastomosis. B) At a later stage, the angiogram shows moderate irrigation of the branches of the middle cerebral artery by the anastomosis. The blood flow continued to be ensured mainly by the collateral circulation via the ophthalmic artery. Due to insufficient flow conditions and a low pressure gradient between the superficial temporal artery and the middle cerebral artery region, there was no postoperative dilatation of the superficial temporal artery 4 weeks postoperatively

extra-intracranial anastomosis is an accurate technique in performing the anastomosis. Stenosis in the anastomotic region will have a seriously adverse effect on the operative results. The so-called "patch technique" according to Koos 1977, provides an extremely wide end-to-side anastomosis and ensures that the postoperative flow will be as good as possible. This technique is described in Chapter 8 (Fig. 62, page 76).

Blood flow is another essential factor affecting the functional performance of a microanastomosis. *If sufficient difference in pressure exists between the extracranial and intracranial circulations, flow will be excellent. This is strongly interrelated with a correct indication for such an operation.* Measurements have shown an average pressure difference of 30 mm Hg between the superficial temporal artery and the cortical artery (Yonekawa 1976). If intracerebral arterial pressure is almost equal to that of the superficial temporal artery, there will be no satisfactory blood flow, and the anastomosis will not function adequately. Therefore, if an intact

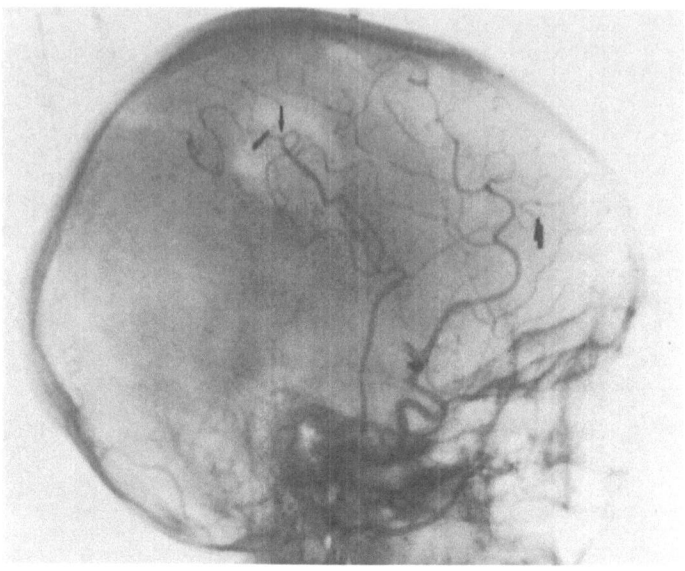

Fig. 36. A 34-year-old female patient with embolic occlusion of the right middle cerebral artery without collateral circulation preoperatively. 7 days, after surgery there was satisfactory dilatation of the superficial temporal artery and there was sufficient irrigation of the angular region by the end-to-side microanastomosis (↑)

vascular system is anastomosed with the extracranial circulation, the danger of anastomotic occlusion is far higher than when a high pressure gradient exists. Thus an operation presents difficulties in regard to stenoses and occlusions. if a very good collateral circulation exists. Case no. 37 in our series (E. K.) showed very good collateral supply in the presence of carotid occlusion. Four weeks after the operation, there was insufficient dilatation of the superficial temporal artery (Fig. 35). A correct indication is thus a precondition for ensuring satisfactory functioning of a microvascular anastomosis; the patient's condition has to require anastomosis. The second important factor in performing the anastomosis is an accurate surgical technique. The superficial temporal artery and the cortical vessel will only be able to dilate to a sufficient extent if these two prerequisites are met. Dilatation of the superficial temporal artery and the cortical vessel then is visible a few days after the operation, as in case 45, a traumatic occlusion of the middle cerebral artery. Eight days postoperatively, satisfactory dilatation of the superficial temporal artery and of the cortical artery can be seen (Fig. 36).

Recanalization of the occluded vessel, as described in Chapter 11.4., is also a factor that may subsequently lead to anastomotic failure.

7. Preoperative Diagnostic Procedures

All authors pay special attention to preoperative diagnostic methods. In reviewing the relevant literature, it becomes obvious that emphasis is laid on angiography, on cerebral blood flow measurement with xenon, and recently on computer tomography as well. This emphasis is understandable considering the fact that routine examinations of patients, particularly those with a cerebral infarction, are taken for granted.

The importance of a detailed history and a routine examination of the patient must be stressed again. In this way transient ischemic attacks and especially their frequency of occurrence can be established. This was pointed out by Chater in 1975 and by Yonekawa and Yaşargil in 1976. Patients seldom report painless symptoms such as transitory dysopia or pareses spontaneously. They must be asked specifically about such symptoms (Marx 1977). As the aim of any surgical procedure is to prevent an imminent attack, it is useful to know that no neurological deficit—which sometimes precedes the attack—has occurred. Other essential symptoms of an insufficient blood supply to the intracranial region are headache or vague dizziness.

7.1. Neurology and Neuropsychology

In addition to a detailed history, all authors also take a careful neurological examination for granted, and thus it is rarely specifically mentioned. This neurological examination, in combination with the patient's history, provides valuable guidelines for a surgical indication, even before the indication for surgery is established by means of other examinations.

The criteria for classifying ischemic cerebral infarction based on the neurological symptoms and the case history are listed in Table 2, where morphological criteria are not taken into account. This classification is commonly used by neurologists and neurosurgeons.

The various stages of cerebrovascular disease combined with morphological findings in general and vascular surgery are outlined in Table 3.

In this author's view, the classification system in Table 3 is not satisfactory, because the morphological change is (incompletely) mentioned only in point 1. Moreover, the term "stages" may give rise to the conclusion that a cerebrovascular disease develops in a series of stages. The classification used in Table 2 is much better; of course, the underlying morphological change must be mentioned separately. The symptoms,

Table 2. *Classification of Ischemic Cerebral Infarction According to Neurological Symptoms and Clinical Development (Without Regard to Morphological Changes)*

Transient Ischemic Attacks (TIA)
Reversible Ischemic Neurological Deficit (RIND)
Prolonged Reversible Ischemic Neurological Deficit (PRIND)
Progressive Stroke (Stroke in Evolution)
Completed Stroke

Table 3. *Classification of Ischemic Cerebral Infarction According to Neurological Symptoms, Clinical Development, and Morphological Changes*

Stage I: asymptomatic stenosis
Stage II: transient ischemic attack
Stage III: progressive stroke
Stage IV: completed stroke

treatment, and prognosis will be dealt with in detail in the relevant chapters.

The neurological examination should also be performed immediately before the operation. This is of particular importance since it is the only method of examination that can be performed again immediately after the operation without straining the patient who has just undergone surgery. At the Department of Neurosurgery, Vienna, it is our practice to have the patient examined by the same neurologist before and after the operation if possible.

Only a few authors mention neuropsychological examination (Chater 1972, Austin 1975, Yonekawa and Yaşargil 1975, Evans and Austin 1977, Holbach 1977). Most of them do not state the type of neuropsychological examination performed, if it was performed at all. It was often observed that the mental activity of the patient improved considerably after such an operation. Yonekawa and Yaşargil 1976 mention that in cases 1 and 6 a state of dementia had greatly improved. Holbach (1977) also reports that in 8 of 11 cases mental avtivity was much better 6 weeks after the operation. Austin (1976) mentions an improved condition in all patients who were monitored psychometrically after the operation. Chater (1977) reports an amelioration of dementia and general activity in the so-called "low-perfusion syndrome".

A few days before surgery 14 patients were given the following series of psychological tests by Evans and Austin (1977): Wechsler Adult Intelligence Scale, Bender Visual-Motor Gestalt Test, Goodenough's Draw a Man Test, and a Proverb Interpretation Test. The tests were repeated 2 to 4 weeks after surgery. A composite score was devised for each patient based on all tests administered to him. Using that total score, it was found that 12 of the 14 patients scored higher after surgery. For 7 of them, the results suggest definite improvement in the intellectual and perceptual motor functions involved.

7.2. EEG

As a preliminary examination, the EEG is very helpful in establishing a differential diagnosis of ischemic cerebral infarction. Although it does not provide a definite differentiation, it may furnish valuable indications. General changes and focal findings in ischemic attacks are rather scarce and usually less pronounced than in hemorrhages or cerebral tumors. A characteristic of such an attack is a discrepancy between the neurological deficiency symptom and slight EEG changes. This can be considered an indication of the formation of ischemia and *vice versa*. EEG monitoring provides valuable clues in differential diagnosis. An involutional process usually sets in a few days after the ischemic attack. After 8 weeks, 40 to 50 percent of the patients still have focal findings, which tend to disappear completely after some time. EEG tracings returning to a normal pattern while the neurological deficit persists one may infer that the cerebral infarction has reached its final stage (cicatricial stage).

Most authors recommend the EEG as a means of preliminary examination, although it is considered a rather unimportant method. In 1975, Yonekawa wrote that "the EEG is of little importance in evaluating the existence of low perfusion in precise ischemic localization". Holbach (1977, case 1) reports EEG changes under *hyperbaric oxygen treatment* and regards the improved EEG as an indication in patients with a completed stroke. An interesting method that might be essential in establishing surgical indication in cases of a completed stroke was described by ITO in 1976. He recorded "evoked potentials" after stimulation of the median nerves in the paralyzed limbs of hemiparetic patients. By using this method, it is easier to evaluate the prognosis of improved neurological symptoms after cerebral revascularization.

7.3. Doppler Sonography

Doppler sonography is based on the shift of frequency observed when a sound source and a receiver are approaching or retreating from each other. It is a highly valuable preliminary diagnostic method in locating suspected stenoses and occlusions in the region of the internal carotid artery. An added advantage to the patient is that it is a painless procedure and it is 90 percent reliable in detecting stenoses and occlusions (Ehringer 1976) in the carotid region. Pathological changes in the carotid region cause a flow reversal in the ophthalmic artery and the frontal artery in the medial orbital corner. The flow reversal observed in this vessel is a reliable and almost consistent pathological finding.

With this method it is only possible to trace stenoses and occlusions in the common carotid artery to the point of bifurcation of the ophthalmic artery from the internal carotid artery. Occlusions and stenoses located distal to this bifurcation are not detectable by Doppler sonography. If manifest neurological deficiency symptoms are present, then a further examination is required.

The most important function of Doppler sonography is to determine the hemodynamic impact of a stenosis in the region of the internal carotid artery. The exact course of the superficial temporal artery can be traced preoperatively.

At the Department of Neurosurgery, Vienna, ultrasonic Doppler sonography is performed on patients suffering from general vascular diseases, even if they do not have neurological symptoms. If the findings are positive, further clarification is obtained by carotid angiography.

7.4. Ophthalmodynamography

This method is an external measurement of the systolic and the diastolic blood pressure of the ophthalmic artery of both eyes and its pulsation volume. A comparison of the results obtained on both sides may reveal unilateral stenoses or occlusions of the carotid arteries.

This method is less reliable than Doppler sonography and fails to produce conclusive data in cases of bilateral occlusions of the internal carotid artery. As in Doppler sonography, it can detect pathological changes in the region of the internal carotid artery only up to the bifurcation of the ophthalmic artery.

7.5. Cerebral Scintigraphy (Brain Scan, Isotope Encephalography)

Cerebral scintigraphy with technetium-99 (^{99}Tc) detects local dysfunction of the blood-brain barrier. Cerebral attacks very seldom produce pathologically increased concentrations of ^{99}Tc during the first 5 days. In the second week after a stroke, findings are positive in 50 to 80 percent of all cases (Marx 1977). After the third week, the concentration of the radioactive indicator decreases, and it is usually no longer detectable 6 to 8 weeks after the attack. This pattern suggests that the concentration of the indicator is linked to repair processes of the cerebral tissue. The regions showing increased concentration correspond more or less to the infarcted areas. Prognostic conclusions cannot be reliably drawn using cerebral scanning as the only method of examination. The amount of concentration of indicator in an area merely indicates the degree of infarction and the prospects of rehabilitation. In regard to reconstructive cerebrovascular surgery, this method is only useful as a means of making a preliminary diagnosis. At best, it may contribute to establishing a differential diagnosis between apoplectic tumors and hemorrhages. This is probably the reason that no author in the literature deals specifically with cerebral scintigraphy with ^{99}Tc. Cerebral scintigraphy with ^{99}Tc has two main advantages. First, it is an aid in locating the ischemic area. Second, it helps to determine the time necessary to complete repair after a completed stroke. Revascularization of the ischemic region may then be performed without causing hemmorrhage or edema.

7.6. Angiography

Angiography of the arteries supplying the brain (four-vessel angiography) is the most important examination method in cerebro-vascular diseases. It is used to establish a differential diagnosis between ischemic lesions and intracranial hemorrhages, brain tumors and malformations of the intracranial vessels. Angiography also provides additional data about the circulation such as direction and velocity of blood flow, as well as data about the collaterals. All authors agree that four-vessel angiography is essential in the detection of cerebrovascular diseases and indications for extra-intracranial anastomosis (Yaşargil 1969, Donaghy 1970, Kikuchi 1972, Reichman 1972, Austin 1974, Heilbrunn 1974, Khodadad 1974, Merei 1974, Weinstein 1974, Gratzl et al. 1975, Spetzler 1975, Yonekawa and Yaşargil 1975, Deruty et al. 1976, Ito 1976—who regards the visualization of the striate arteries as particularly important, Schmiedek et al. 1976, Holbach 1977, Stephens 1977, Thompson et al. 1977).

The technique of cerebral angiography is so well known that no further description is necessary. Nonetheless, it should be mentioned that a constant flow of the contrast medium must be maintained and that angiography must be performed simultaneously in two planes.

The use of insufficient equipment must be absolutely avoided. This increases the hazards to the patient considerably and reduces the diagnostic value of the method. The diagnostic value of angiography may be improved with magnification and with photographic or electronic erasure of superimposed bone structures.

An accurate indication for surgery on the supplying cerebral vessels can be established either extracranially—for example, by endarterectomy of the common carotid artery or the internal carotid artery—or by extra-intracranial anastomosis. The visualization of all afferent and all intracranial vessels is absolutely necessary. Four-vessel angiography can reveal the following:

1. location of the cerebrovascular lesion,
2. degree of the stenosis or the occlusion,
3. existence of multiple lesions,
4. existence and degree of collateral circulation,
5. course and size of the superficial temporal artery or occipital artery to determine the donor vessel.

Angiography can also establish an indication for extra-intracranial bypass by detecting the following pathological changes:

1. occlusion of the internal carotid artery or the common carotid artery,

2. stenosis of the internal carotid artery in the intracranial part,
3. occlusion of the middle cerebral artery,
4. stenosis of the middle cerebral artery,
5. multiple occlusions and stenoses in the carotid and vertebrobasilar regions,
6. occlusions and stenoses in the vertebrobasilar region,
7. operations that may cause a lesion of a large cerebral vessel, such as tumors, aneurysms, and angiomas,
8. moya-moya.

For details see Chapter 11.

If angiography is performed several weeks prior to the operation, follow-up angiography should be performed in the area of the lesion immediately before the operation. This is of particular importance because cerebrovascular lesions occasionally disappear within a short period of time, as demonstrated by the following case:

An 18-year-old female patient was admitted to the hospital with a lefthemisphere stroke, high-grade rightside paresis, and almost complete aphasia. She presented the following risk factors: high-grade adiposity, nicotine abuse, and contraceptive medication.

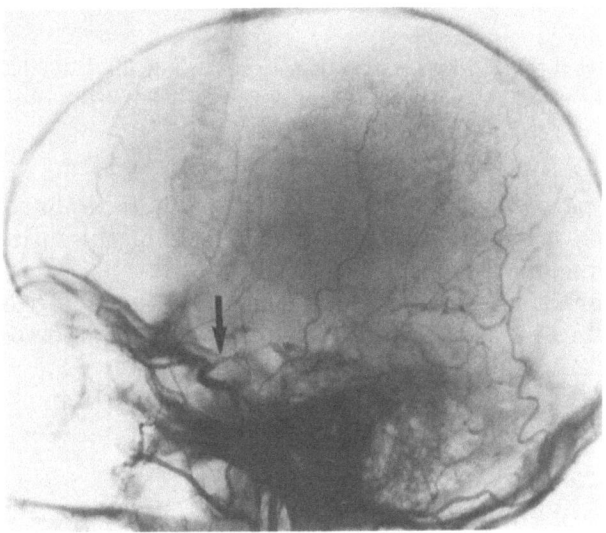

Fig. 37. Angiogram of a 18-year-old female who experienced sudden right sided paresis accompanied by an almost complete aphasia. The angiogram shows an occlusion of the internal carotid artery in the intracranial region just before the bifurcation

The angiography showed an occlusion of the internal carotid artery near the intracranial bifurcation (Fig. 37). Because of the severe, neurological findings, the operation was scheduled to take place 5 weeks after the stroke. In the meantime, routine examinations, such a Doppler sonography, cerebral scintigraphy, cerebral blood flow measurement with xenon, and computerized tomography, were performed, The clinical status improved slightly. Carotid angiography was again performed on the left side 1 day before the scheduled operation. The angiogram showed patency at the site of the previous occlusion (Fig. 38). Thus surgery was no longer indicated.

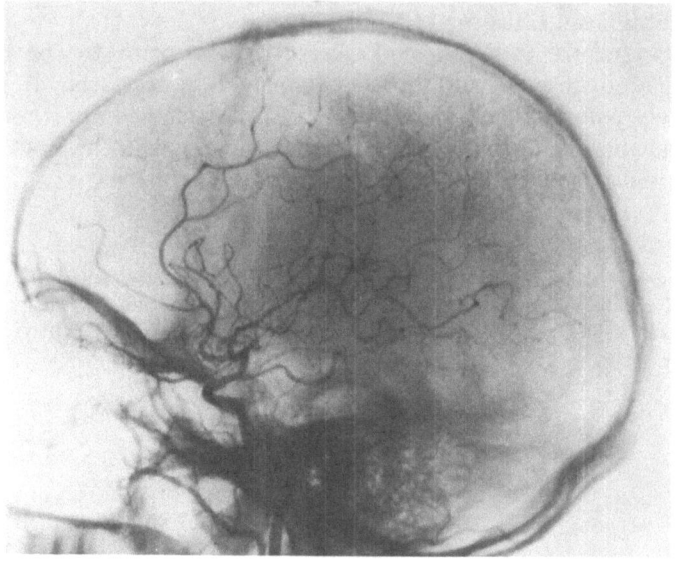

Fig. 38. Angiogram taken 5 weeks after that shown in Fig. 38, 1 day before the extra-intracranial bypass operation was scheduled. Recanalization can be seen at the previously occluded site

Over the past 3 years in more than 20 patients we have observed a recanalization of occluded or stenosed vessels in the intracranial and extracranial regions (see also Chapter 11.4.).

The examination scheme used at the Department of Neurosurgery, Vienna, to detect indications for extra-intracranial anastomosis following stroke or T.I.A. is described on page 115 and 122.

Postoperative angiography is also extremely important in the evaluation of the results of an operation.

7.7. Regional Cerebral Blood Flow Measurement

Over the last 30 years, there has been growing interest in the physiology of cerebral blood flow (CBF). This was brought about by the development of new quantitative methods. In 1945, Kety and Schmidt introduced the nitrous oxide method as an invasive quantitative technique for measuring global CBF. This method is accurate from a qualitative point of view and does not require puncture of the internal carotid artery. Its disadvantage is that only global and not regional CBF (rCBF) measurement is obtained.

Other nonquantitative methods of clinical interest, such as sequential scintiphotography (Heiss *et al*. 1972), intravenous technitium angiography (Planiol *et al*. 1971), or intracarotid radioactive microsphere angiography (Blaudino 1973), are also being used to study disturbances in brain perfusion, especially in patients with anomalies of the large extracranial arteries.

For a more detailed and comprehensive analysis of the physiopathology of CBF, the reader is referred to reviews such as those by Lassen (1959), Sokoloff (1959), Beth (1972), Moosmann (1974), Olesen (1974), and Herrschaft (1975).

The method for measurement of rCBF with radioactive inert gases was proposed by Lassen and Ingvar in 1961. Its principle is the assumption that the removal of a freely diffusible and inert indicator from a tissue is a function of the perfusion rate of that tissue. If one uses radioactive γ-emitting isotopes as indicators, it is then possible to record the clearance from various areas of the brain through the intact cranium by multiple detectors placed over the patient's scalp.

The radioactive gas originally used was krypton ([84]Kr). Its radioactive characteristics permit a good counting efficiency because of the high energy of its γ radiations (0.5 MeV). The physical half-life of this isotope, however, is rather long, 10.5 years, and only 0.4 percent of its emissions are in the form of γ rays.

Because of these disadvantages investigators have turned to another radioactive inert gas, xenon-133 (^{133}Xe).

From the data recorded from the samples, rCBF can be calculated in several ways: 1. compartmental analysis (Lassen *et al*. 1963); 2. stochastic analysis (Zierler 1965); and 3. initial slope analysis (Hoedt-Rasmussen 1967).

The ^{133}Xe clearance method has the advantage of measuring regional and global CBF simultaneously with sufficient accuracy. The global CBF measurement is obtained by calculating the average value. An approximate calculation can be performed separately for gray and white matter. A major disadvantage of this method is the necessary injection of ^{133}Xe into the internal carotid artery. To avoid intra-arterial injection, experiments have been performed using the inhalation of [133]Xe. However, the extracerebral presence of the isotope is an inconvenience caused by these methods.

Extra-intracranial bypass improves flow in strictly defined ischemic areas. Medical centers that practice this procedure have dealt intensively with this examination method both preoperatively and postoperatively (Austin 1974, 1975, Heilbrunn 1974, Gratzl *et al*. 1975, Reichmann 1975, Schmiedek and Gratzl 1976, and Ito *et al*. 1976, who also performed rCBF measurements during the operation).

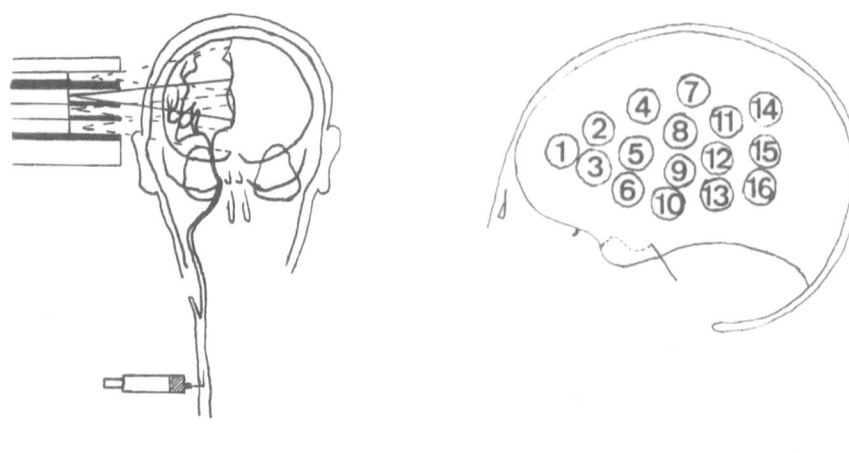

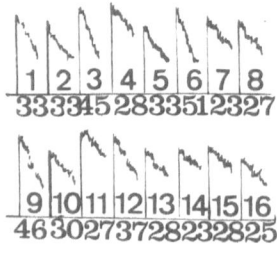

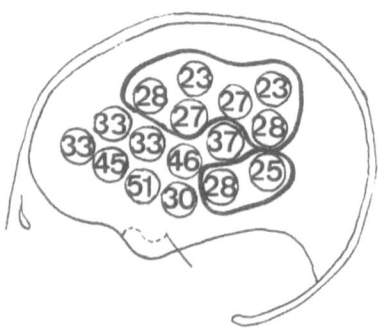

Fig. 39. rCBF measured with 133 Xe in 16 regions. The evaluation of the curves is limited to the initial 2 minutes. Further reduction of the size of probes allows rCBF to be measured in up to 35 regions. Use of a small digital computer on-line gives the rCBF values per unit time along with a graphic representation of the regions with decreased blood flow

Schmiedek *et al.* (1976) wrote that "measurement of rCBF allows the clinician for the first time to assess the objective flow abnormalities present in a patient with ischemic cerebrovascular disease. The rCBF results not only allow a classification of patients with selection of those most likely to benefit from surgery, but this method also localizes the cortical ischemic areas into which extracranial vessel should be anastomosed".

The postoperative occlusion of a vessel can be prevented by a low-pressure gradient because flow in an ischemic area can be accurately determined by means of this method (Chapter 6). Schmiedek reported in

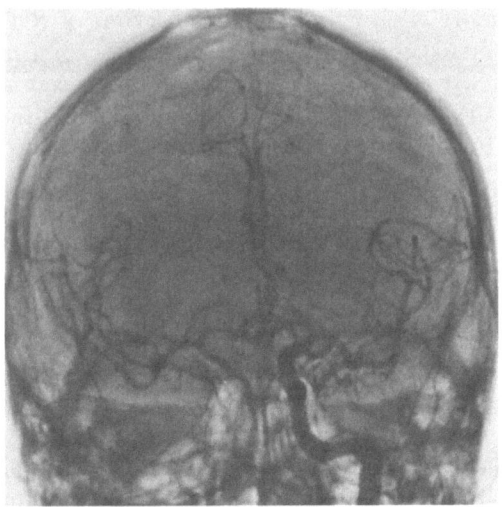

Fig. 40. Angiogram of a 59-year-old patient with a right sided carotid occlusion and ideal crossflow from the left to the right. CBF measurement with 133 Xe revealed only an insignificant reduction in CBF, so that extra-intracranial anastomosis was not required. The patient recieves regular check-ups

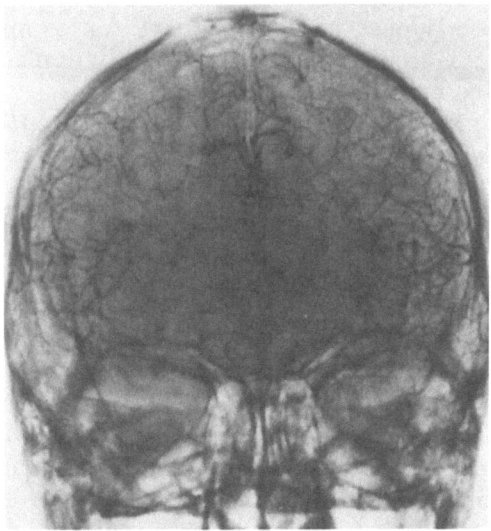

Fig. 41. Late phase of the angiogram shown in Fig. 40 shows a balanced supply to both brain hemispheres in the capillaries

1976 that "in all patients with TIA and clearly reduced rCBF, postoperative angiography revealed patency of the anastomosis, "on the other hand, patients with generalized reduction of rCBF, who show no clinical improvement and a high occlusion rate of the bypass, do not appear to benefit from the extra-intracranial arterial bypass".

Some authors regard "clinical and angiographical findings as the only decisive criteria for indication of this operation" (Chater 1974, Yonekawa and Yaşargil 1976).

This method is undoubtedly a valuable aid in assessing the advisability of extra-intracranial anastomosis whenever the extent of CBF decrease is not precisely known. This may be the case in a patient without neurological deficit who complains of transient ischemic attacks and whose angiogram shows a clear morphological substrate—for example a carotid occlusion—with ideal collateral circulation. Figures 40 and 41 show the angiogram of a patient with rightside carotid occlusion and ideal cross flow. This patient's history revealed three TIA. CBF measurements showed a very slight decrease in CBF in both hemispheres; therefore, extra-intracranial anastomosis was not performed. Neurological findings in this patient have been normal for about 1 year and his condition is checked regularly.

Thus rCBF measurement has essentially the following three advantages:

1. Accurate localization of the ischemic area provides the correct localization of the anastomosis.

2. It is an additional aid in cases where clinical and angiographic findings alone are insufficient to determine whether there is low perfusion.

3. It provides evidence of postoperative functioning of the extra-intracranial anastomosis because an irreversibly damaged brain cannot show postoperative increase of rCBF.

It must be emphasized, however, that the rCBF method can hardly be employed on a routine base in the preoperative evaluation of all potential candidates for bypass surgery.

7.8. Computerized Tomography

Computerized axial scanning (Computerized axial tomography–CAT scan) is an exciting noninvasive radiological technique with which, in effect, a soft tissue tomographic view of the brain is obtained in the transverse axial plane (Hounsfield 1973).

Differences in tissue density are an indication of underlying pathological processes. Processes accompanied by increased density (sclerosis, meningioma, fresh hemorrhage, etc.) can be clearly differentiated from those associated with reduced density (cerebral edema, cerebral infarction, cysts, etc.). In cerebroatrophic processes, ventricular and subarachnoid enlargement can be visualized. The evidence provided by this method can be further enhanced by intravenous injection of a contrast medium containing iodine.

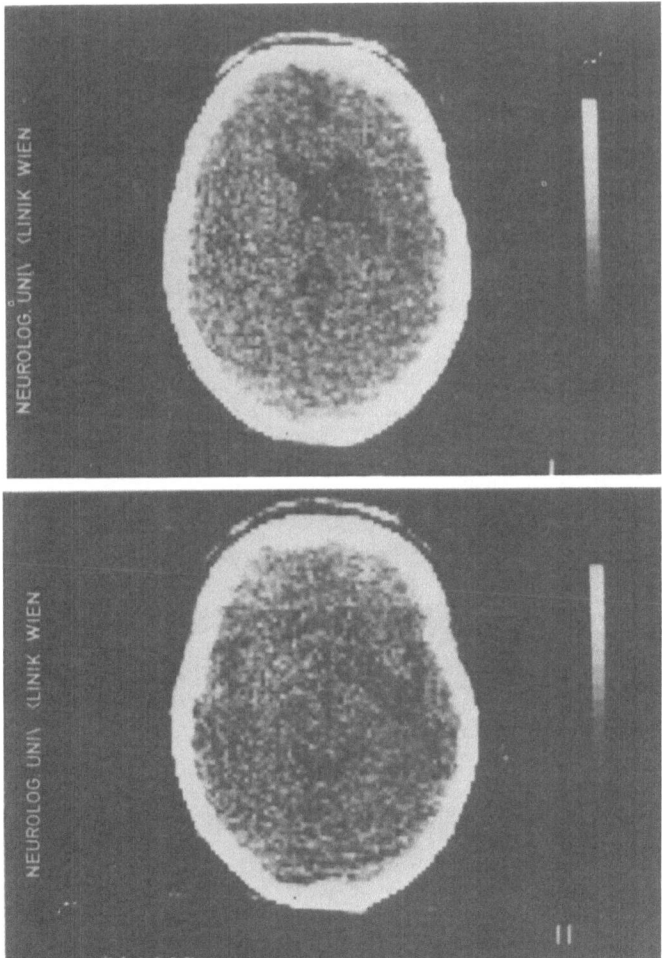

Fig. 42. Computerized tomogram of a 65-year-old patient with right sided carotid occlusion. A medium-grade density reduction can be seen in the right hemisphere. Reduced density is also visible in the central region on the left side. This condition is a very good indication for an extra-intracranial bypass

One of the most useful roles for this unique development will be its ability, without danger to the patient, to distinguish between cerebral infarction and cerebral hemorrhage in the early days after a stroke. This method is atraumatic; radiation exposure per layer corresponds to that of a cranial x-ray.

Since it is a relatively recent method, only some of the authors dealing with extra-intracranial anastomosis have sufficient experience to give a definite assessment of its diagnostic value.

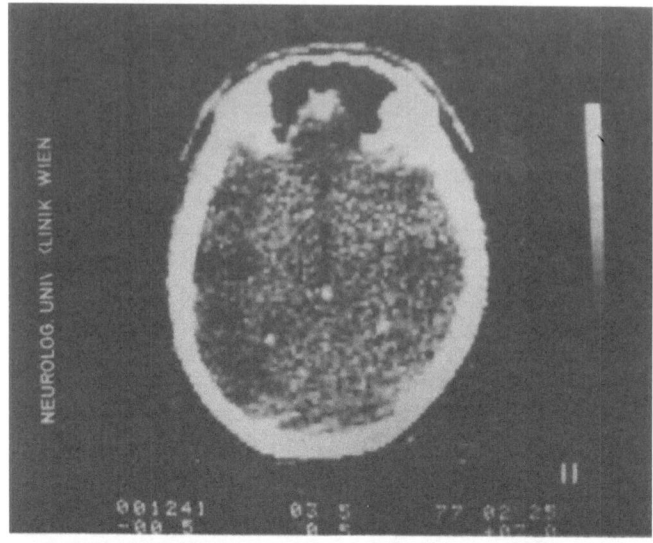

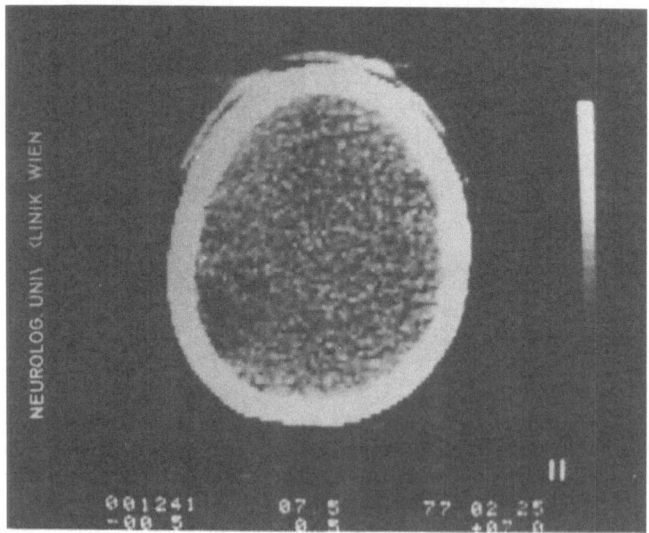

Fig. 43. Computerized tomogram of a 63-year-old patient with a carotid occlusion on the left and a large-scale density reduction in the left hemisphere, accompanied by the formation of small cysts, particularly in the parieto-occipital region. There is also a slight density reduction on the right in the temporoparietal region. This condition is a good indication for surgery, although a complete restitution of the neurological deficits cannot be expected

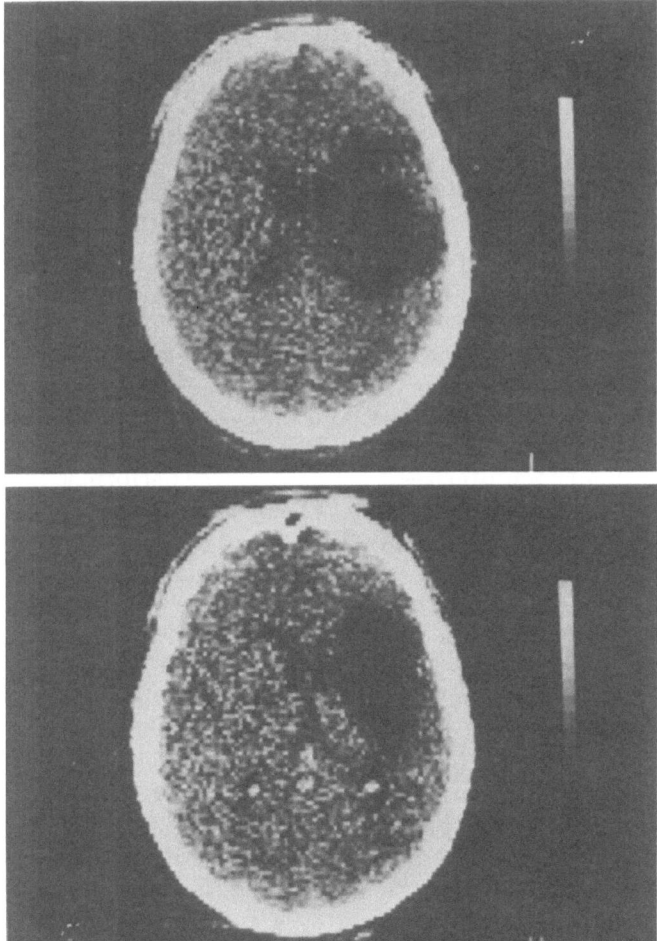

Fig. 44. Occlusion of the right middle cerebral artery (*MCA*) in a 34-year-old female patient. There is a large cyst formation in the MCA region on the right. In this case, vascular reconstruction cannot improve the neurological symptoms

At the second Symposium on Cerebrovascular Diseases, Davis reported on the use of computerized tomography in acute stroke. In 1975, Hounsfield published a comprehensive study on computerized tomography and the management of cerebrovascular disease. Up to that time, mainly the size and location of affected areas and edema could be traced by this method. In 1975, Yonekawa wrote that "it is not possible to detect an area of low perfusion with this method so far".

This limitation still remains for TIA or low perfusion not followed by a pathological substrate. However, particularly in the case of manifest neurological deficit, computerized tomography provides relatively satisfactory evidence of the extent of parenchymatous damage. In completed stroke, it can thus be decided whether surgery is advisable or not.

If the density in an ischemic area is slightly or severely reduced, revascularization is indicated (Fig. 42, 43). On the other hand, complete parenchymatous atrophy associated with the formation of cysts is a contraindication to extra-intracranial bypass (Fig. 44). This applies particularly to strokes that occurred some time ago and have caused persistent manifest neurological deficit. In 1975, Gratzl reported on seven patients with slight or severe generalized reduction in rCBF which did not improve at all postoperatively. At that time, computerized tomography was not yet performed. There was apparently massive damage to the parenchyma that could not be detected by any method available at that time. Schmiedek and Gratzl (1976) reported on two patients in whom computerized tomography was performed in addition to rCBF studies. In case 1 the computer tomogram showed a large infarction on the left side with extensive involvement of a region normally supplied by the middle cerebral artery. As the patient had a normal rCBF study, the decision was made not to operate.

The major advantage of computerized tomography is the fact that it can be repeated within a short period of time and that it is a painless procedure. Computerized tomography is also feasible immediately after the operation. Figure 45 shows the tomogram of a 54-year-old patient in whom a hemorrhage was suspected in the anastomotic region after extra-intracranial bypass. However, a large cerebral edema was detected, so that no further operation was performed.

A second advantage is that this technique is the only one that reliably detects necroses and severe loss of tissue substance. Thus surgery can be excluded in certain patients.

Furthermore, differential diagnosis between tumors and hemorrhages is easily feasible. Another advantage is that only problem cases (such as case 2 described by Schmiedek in 1976) have to be submitted to additional tests, for example, rCBF measurement.

Only in recent times has computerized tomography become part of the preoperative diagnostic battery for extra-intracranial anastomosis (Schmiedek et al. 1978, Spetzler et al. 1978). For this reason, the value of this technique, particularly for selection of patients with a completed stroke, cannot be definitely assessed. According to the experience at the Department of Neurosurgery, Vienna, we think that computerized tomography is a very decisive indication of the operability of the patient. Its diagnostic value is secondbest after that of angiography, and an excellent clinical-anatomic correlation was obtained by computerized tomography in all cases in which cerebral ischemia had led to morphological alterations of the brain tissue, such as in patients with completed stroke and those in the PRIND group. Based on the localization and the extent of the infarction, the following five groups of

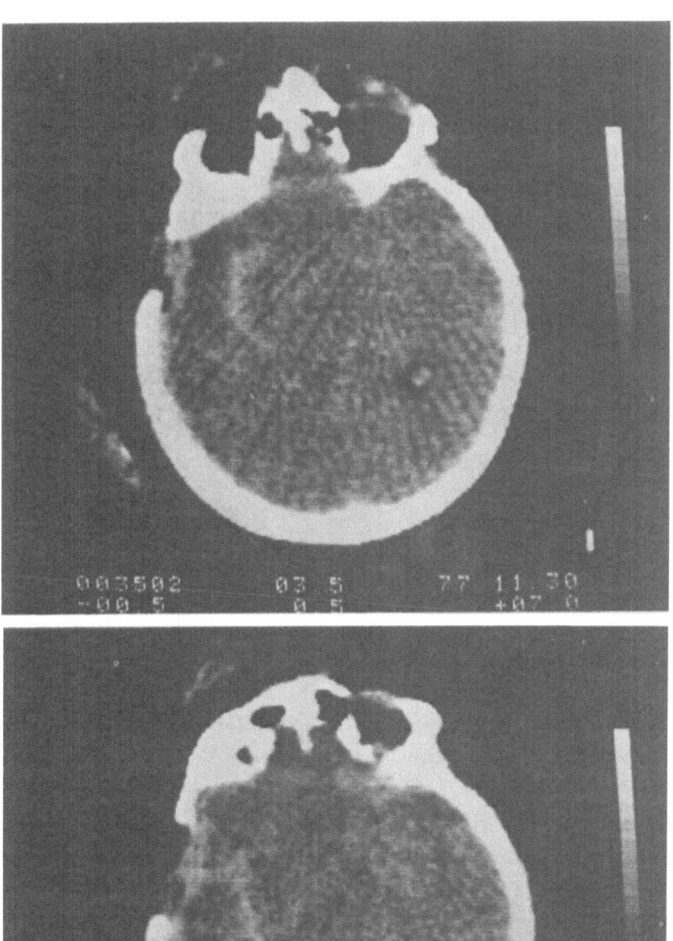

Fig. 45. Computerized tomogram of a 54-year-old patient (case 76) with carotid occlusion 5 hours after extra-intracranial bypass operation on the left. Immediately after the operation, the patient was in a comatose state, with massive right sided hemiplegia. Because intracranial bleeding was suspected, computerized tomography was performed postoperatively. It clearly revealed a bony lesion at the site of anastomosis, as well as considerable cerebral edema, particularly in the left hemisphere. The ventricular system was seen only on the right side. There was only little blood in the sylvian fossa, which does not, however, account for the massive symptoms. No revision was performed on the evidence of the computerized tomogram

computerized tomographic abnormalities can be differentiated in patients with cerebrovascular disease:

1. Normal scan (in cases of TIA and RIND),

2. Relatively small infarction localized within the subcortical region (PRIND and CS),

3. Cortical infarction involving only a section of the MCA and usually surrounded by a boundary zone with varying tissue absorption values (CS),

4. Deep small infarction within the internal capsule (so-called "strategic infarction"),

5. Massive infarction.

For the last two findings on operation is not indicated by the computerized tomographic evidence.

7.9. Conclusion

Although all the preoperative examination methods described are of great importance and are desirable for the indication of a bypass operation, in most cases it is sufficient to record the patient's detailed history and neurological condition and to perform four-vessel angiography.

By using the most important techniques, described above, selection of patients for surgery is also practicable in small hospitals that do not have all the existing methods of examination (such as computerized tomography) at their disposal (Stephens 1977, Zumstein 1977).

Preliminary diagnostic studies include principally EEG, Doppler sonography, and scintigraphy. If these tests reveal that a lesion of the afferent cerebral arteries may be suspected, further examinations, such as angiography and computerized tomography, are necessary.

In problem cases, however—this applies particularly to TIA patients without angiographically detectable lesions or patients with a completed stroke—detailed examinations, including rCBF measurement and computerized tomography, are absolutely required (Chapters 11 and 12).

In this author's opinion, more attention should be paid to pre- and postoperative neuropsychological and psychiatric tests. At present, there are not enough methods providing objective evidence of a psychiatric and psychological improvement, particularly in the low-perfusion syndrome. However, many authors mention a generally improved mental condition in many patients.

8. Timing of the Operation

It is surprising that the available literature rarely refers to the optimal timing of the operation. Gratzl (1975) is absolutely against surgery for traumatic vascular occlusions within the first hours after the trauma. This view is shared by Chater (1976), who had a postoperative fatality after surgery in the acute phase. Figures 98–103 show the angiogram of a patient after an extra-intracranial anastomosis operation for a left-sided carotid occlusion. Shortly after the operation the right carotid artery occluded. Twenty-four hours later, an extra-intracranial bypass was performed on the recent right carotid occlusion. This patient died of a massive cerebral edema 5 days after the second operation. Only one case has been described in the relevant literature (Yaşargil 1970, case 2) in which extra-intracranial anastomosis was performed 3 days after aneurysm surgery and completed stroke after operation. This patient made a very rapid postoperative recovery.

Holbach (1976) suggests that the optimal time for surgery in completed stroke is 4 weeks after the acute trauma. Hitl (1976) usually waits 3 weeks before performing the operation in order to see whether or not conservative treatment improves the patient's condition. Irino (1976) also recommends waiting a while for recanalization.

In this author's opinion, *surgery within the first 2 weeks after a stroke is absolutely inadvisable*. Hypoxemia impairs the function of the blood-brain barrier. This usually results in a massive cerebral edema whenever revascularization is performed, and invariably results in the patient's death. Bleeding into the infarcted area is occasionally provoked and causes a serious deterioration in the patient's condition. This has also been described in relation to surgery on the cervical vessels.

Our experience with completed strokes shows that *the optimal time for the operation is 4-6 weeks* after the stroke (Tables 4 and 11, pages 60 and 124).

Surgery is also feasible as early as 20 days after the event, since the blood-brain barrier function is stabilized by then. *Surgery may even be performed up to 3 months* after the stroke. A good recovery was achieved in only a few cases after this length of time (Table 11, page 124).

In cases of transient ischemic attacks, surgery should be carried out as soon as possible (see also Chapter 12.1) after angiography. In doubtful cases angiography should be supplimented by rCBF measurement with xenon and computerized tomography. One should always anticipate a manifest stroke, which occurs in an average of 40 to 50 percent of the cases within 1 year (Fischer 1951, 1959; Fields *et al*. 1970) (see Table 11, page 124).

Table 4. *Optimal and Good Timing for Extra-Intracranial Anastomosis-Procedure*

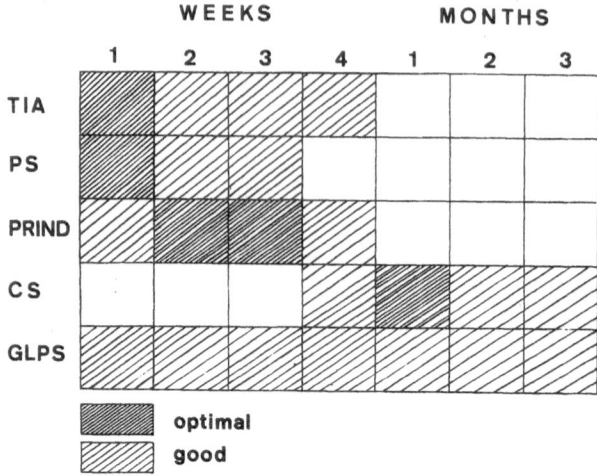

On the basis of the clinical results of vascular surgery for *rapid progressive stroke* (see Chapter 12.4.), surgery in these cases is contraindicated. In cases of *slow progressive stroke*, extra-intracranial anastomosis is *indicated as soon as possible*.

The *generalized low-perfusion syndrome* deserves, in this author's opinion, to be emphasized in the whole pattern of completed stroke. Contraindications for operation are shown in Table 5.

Table 5. *Contraindications*

Unconsciousness
Major strokes with severe neurological deficits
Cerebral edema
Diffuse cerebral occlusive disease
Other severe diseases (cardiopulmonary, cancer etc.)

9. Operative Technique

Pre- and postoperative care of the patient as well as anesthesia are performed according to general practice in neurosurgery and need not be treated specifically in this study. The operation itself requires the use of some special instruments (Fig. 46) and the operating microscope. The exposure of the superficial temporal artery is sometimes possible without the operating microscope and is a technique preferred by some neurosurgeons. For the exposure of the cortical vessels, however, sufficient magnification (25 to 40 times) is absolutely necessary. The suturing of a satisfactory anastomosis is also not feasible without an operating microscope. The prerequisites for acquiring the microsurgical technique, particularly microsurgical exposure of small vessels and suturing of microanastomoses, are discussed in Chapter 5. The operative technique employed worldwide was introduced by Yaşargil and Donaghy in 1967. Although some modifications have been developed, the principle remains the same: *establishment of an artificial collateral circulation between the branches of the external carotid artery and the internal carotid artery* (Fig. 47, page 63).

For more than 10 years the superficial temporal artery or the occipital artery hase been used as the afferent branch of extra-intracranial anastomoses. These arteries have shown excellent suitability (Yaşargil 1969, Reichmann 1972, Kletter *et al.* 1975). Practical experience has also shown that the interposition of prosthetic grafts, veins, or arteries is not suitable.

The author's own experience has shown that arteries, f.e., the radial artery, have a strong spasmophilic tendency. It is this characteristic feature that makes an occlusion of the anastomosis highly probable if the radial artery is used as an implant. Despite intensive experimental studies undertaken on a worldwide scale, it has been shown that the superficial temporal artery cannot be satisfactorily replaced by any vein, artery, or autogenous graft.

An average patency rate of 80 to 90 percent has been found in the cases in which there was correct indication and correct surgical technique (Ausman 1972, Austin 1972, Piepgras 1972, Reichmann 1972, Chater 1976, Peerless 1976). The duration of the operation is of some importance, considering that it has to be performed by means of a microsurgical technique. This operation usually takes 6 hours (Acland 1976), although sometimes it takes less than 4 hours.

On the basis of the existing literature it is difficult to conclude if the use of anticoagulants, such as heparin, is advisable. Although the use of heparin is sometimes mentioned, anticoagulant substances do not seem to be commonly used. At the Department of Neurosurgery, Vienna, no anticoagulant was used in any of the operations performed thus far.

9.1. Exposure of the Superficial Temporal Artery

The patient is placed on his back, with his head turned sideward (Fig. 48). The branches of the external carotid artery to be anastomosed

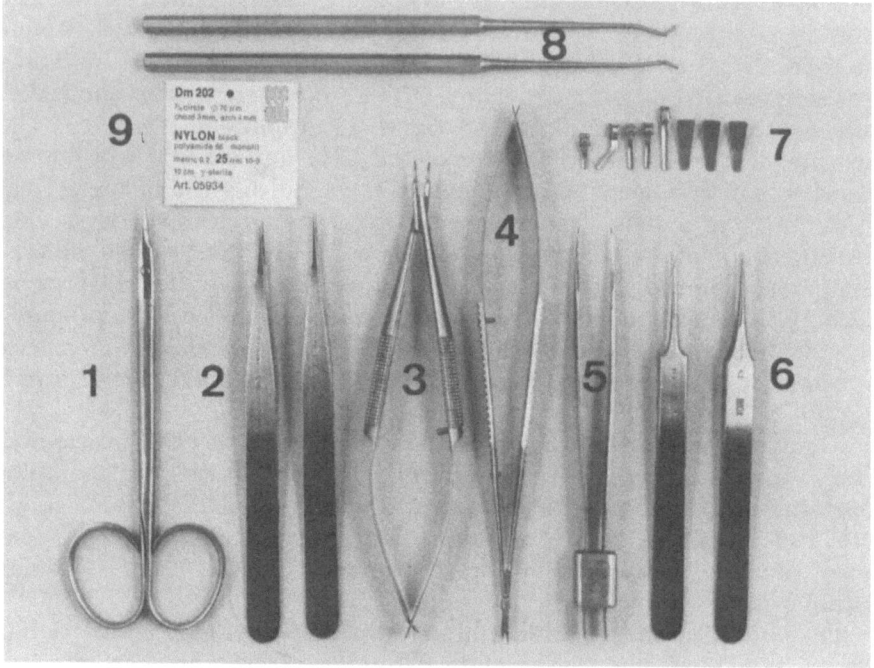

Fig. 46. Special instruments used in extra-intracranial anastomosis: Microscissors (1, 4); microforceps (2, 5, 6); needleholder (3); microdissectors (8); microclamps (7); 10/0 microsutures (9)

have to be checked angiographically in regard to their course and actual suitability, prior to the operation. Chater (1976) considers an all too thin superficial temporal artery as a contraindication for this operation. This author does not share his opinion and believes that if the indication for surgery is correct and the operation is performed adequately, the superficial temporal artery, however thin it may be, can always dilate to a certain extent. A superselective visualization of the external carotid artery can be performed additionally with a catheter if necessary.

The original method, according to Yaşargil, consists of a semicircular incision situated in such a way that the branches of the superficial temporal artery are more or less in its center (Fig. 49).

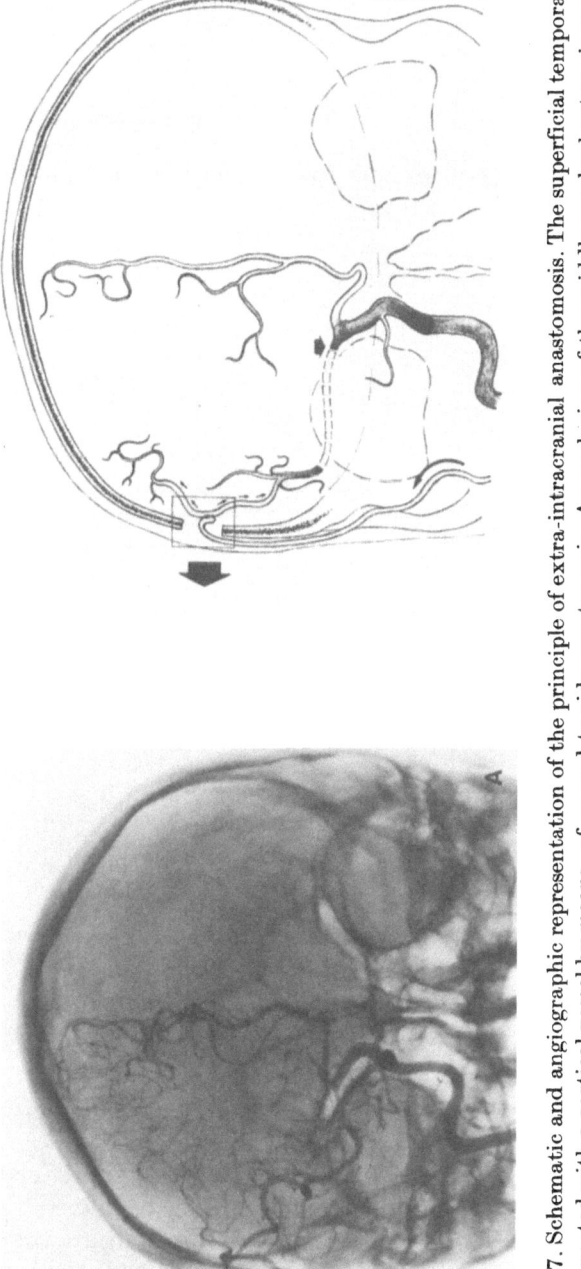

Fig. 47. Schematic and angiographic representation of the principle of extra-intracranial anastomosis. The superficial temporal artery is connected with a cortical vessel by means of an end-to-side anastomosis. An occlusion of the middle cerebral artery is used as an example

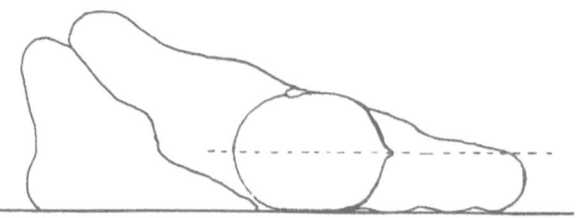

Fig. 48. Patient's position on the operating table (according to kempe)

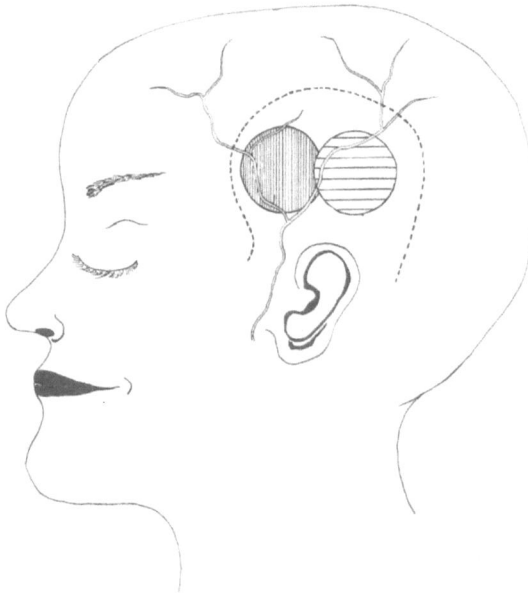

Fig. 49. Exposure of the superficial temporal artery as the skin flap is formed. If possible, the parietal and frontal branches of the superficial temporal artery should be situated more or less in the center part of the flap

The arteries that bleed and pulsate from the skin incision can be ligated or closed by small clamps. Such ligatures or clamps can be used to indicate the prospective direction and course of the superficial temporal artery in the skin flap, though the latter is not yet visible. The skin flap is reflected carefully with blunt dissection so as not to injure the superficial temporal artery. The pulsation of the superficial temporal artery distinguishes it from concomitant veins (Fig. 50).

It is advisable to start exposing the superficial temporal artery proximally at its trunk to facilitate the technical procedure.

The superficial temporal artery is dissected from the inferior surface of the scalp flap (Fig. 51). Difficulties may arise in the case of a slightly indurated galea if the patient's history includes skull injuries. Furthermore, arterial loops occur to a considerable extent in severe arteriosclerosis. The number of vessel loops increases with the patient's advancing age to the same extent as cerebral sclerosis (see Figs. 2-6). This is obviously due to the pathological and anatomical characteristics of the

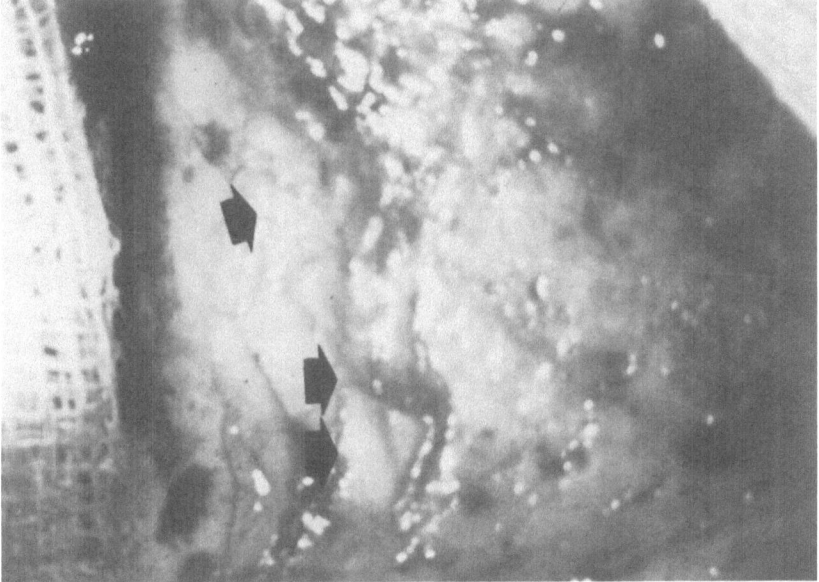

Fig. 50. After the skin flap is retracted, the superficial temporal artery is rarely visible but can be traced by palpation. The vessel (arrows) is clearly visible after the fascia is opened

superficial temporal artery (Lie *et al.* 1970, Sinzinger *et al.* 1975, Kletter *et al.* 1976, 1977). A relatively large branch coming off the apex of each loop can be expected to be found during exposure. These branches can be either coagulated or, if they are very large, ligated with 0-6 or 0-7 suture material in order to prevent thrombus formation due to clotting (Fig. 52).

In order to prevent postoperative complications, a sufficiently large fibrous mantle should be left around the vessel. This protective cover enables the surgeon to handle the vessel without injuring the vessel wall and guarantees improved nutrition of the vessels of the external carotid region. After completing the exposure, a rubber foil should be placed under the artery (Fig. 51).

According to Peerless (1977), it is also possible to dissect the superficial temporal artery with an incision exactly above the vessel, whose course

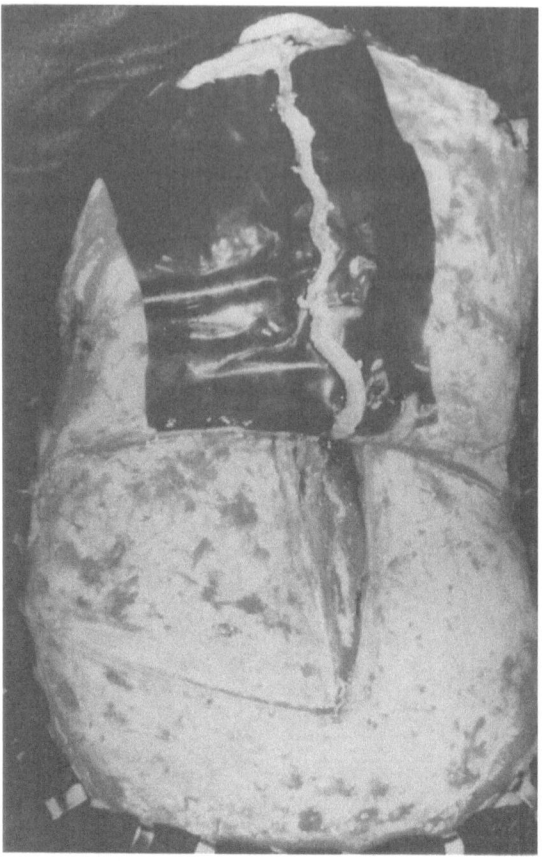

Fig. 51. A piece of rubber glove is placed under the vessel after the exposure of the
superficial temporal artery. Large branches coming off the artery have been ligated;
smaller branches have been closed by bipolar coagulation. The temporal muscle is then
incised, and a burr hole is made and enlarged

has been previously traced by palpation, angiography and, when possible,
echography (Fig. 53). This direct exposure of the superficial temporal
artery without a skin flap allows a better blood supply to the scalp. Some
authors consider the use of both main branches of the superficial temporal
artery (frontal and parietal) as advantageous, improving the perfusion of
the region to be anastomosed (Fig. 54). When both branches of the
superficial temporal artery are used, the risk of a scalp necrosis is
particularly great.

However, it has been observed that the capacity of the superficial
temporal artery is dependent on its main trunk. Thus, if this vessel dilates
to only twice its original diameter, the blood flow passing through it will
be four times as high (Spetzler and Chater 1976, Kletter *et al.* 1975, 1976).

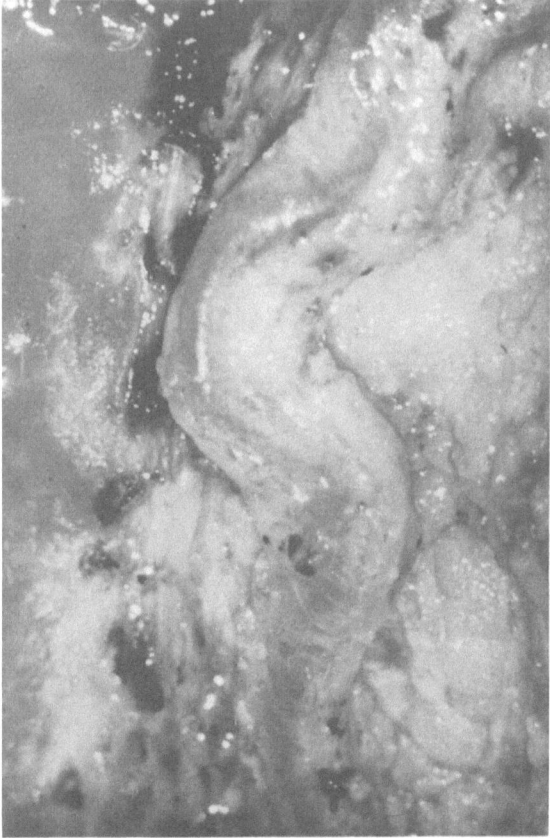

Fig. 52. A large meandering of the superficial temporal artery is an indication of rather severe arteriosclerosis. A large vessel may be expected to bifurcate on the outer side of every loop

The next step is to severe the temporal muscle. This is usually done in the form of an inverse T or L (Fig. 51). This muscle incision, either angular or temporal, must take into account the region to be supplied by the anastomosis. After reflecting the incised muscle, an enlarged burr hole of about 3×3 cm is usually sufficient. A bone flap is necessary if it is not clear preoperatively whether cortical vessels are to be found in the target region. This procedure may also be used for other reasons, such as operations for vessel malformations or tumors in which external-internal anastomoses are necessary (Chapter 11).

Exposure of the occipital artery

The exposure of this vessel at the inner surface of the scalp flap is impeded by the overlapping occipital muscle. Palpation of the artery is

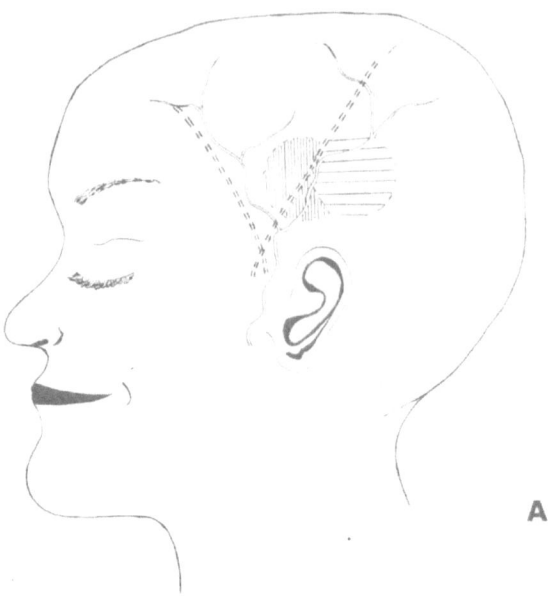

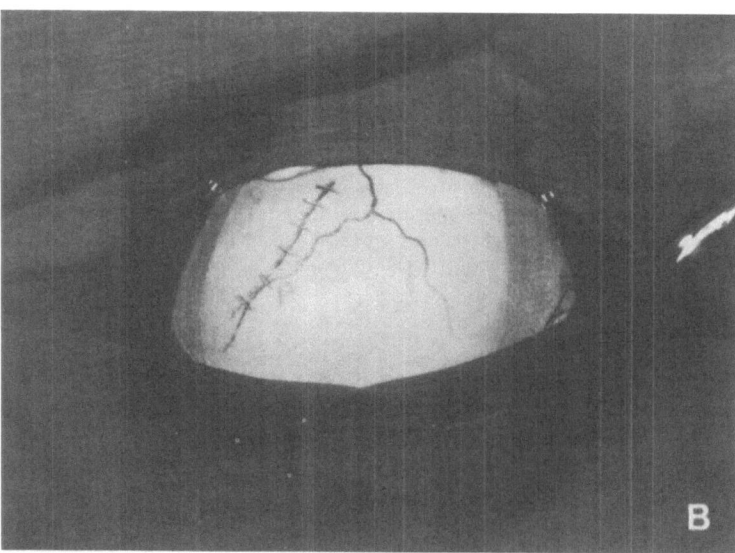

Fig. 53. Direct exposure of the superficial temporal artery with a skin incision. The path of the vessel is checked preoperatively by either palpation or ultrasonic measurement

extremely difficult or even impossible because of the relatively massive muscle layer and the fascia. Usually it is necessary to dissect free a rather long portion of the occipital artery (Fig. 8 A, page 14).

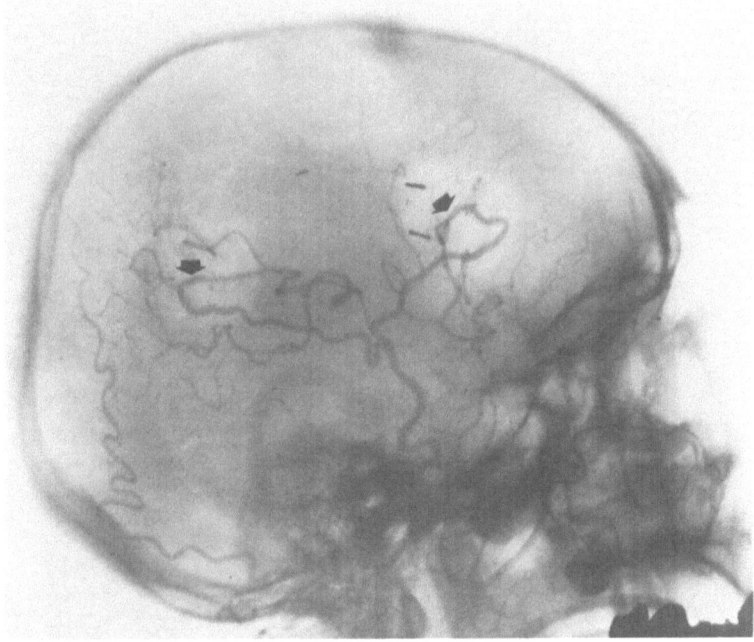

Fig. 54. In special cases both branches can be used for the extra-intracranial anastomosis. Good supply to the cortical vessel with the well-functioning anastomoses (arrows) can be seen

9.2. Exposure of the Cortical Vessel

After opening of the dura crosswise, the surgeon attempts to identify a suitable cortical vessel. This is sometimes difficult, because the cortical vessels are surrounded by a thickened arachnoid in patients with a stroke. Large veins can also be concomitant to the cortical artery (Fig. 55). An appropriate cortical vessel, which should have a diameter of not less than 0.6 to 0.8 mm, will frequently not be found in this 3 × 3 cm burr hole. A cortical vessel of smaller dimensions is unsuitable for anastomosis. The smaller the vessel is, the higher the rate of occlusion of the microanastomoses (Chater 1976, Yonekawa and Yaşargil 1976).

Chater *et al.* studied 40 brains and made accurate measurements of the diameter of the vessels branching from the middle cerebral artery and coursing along the cortex. Figure 56 reveals that in a 4-cm diameter bony

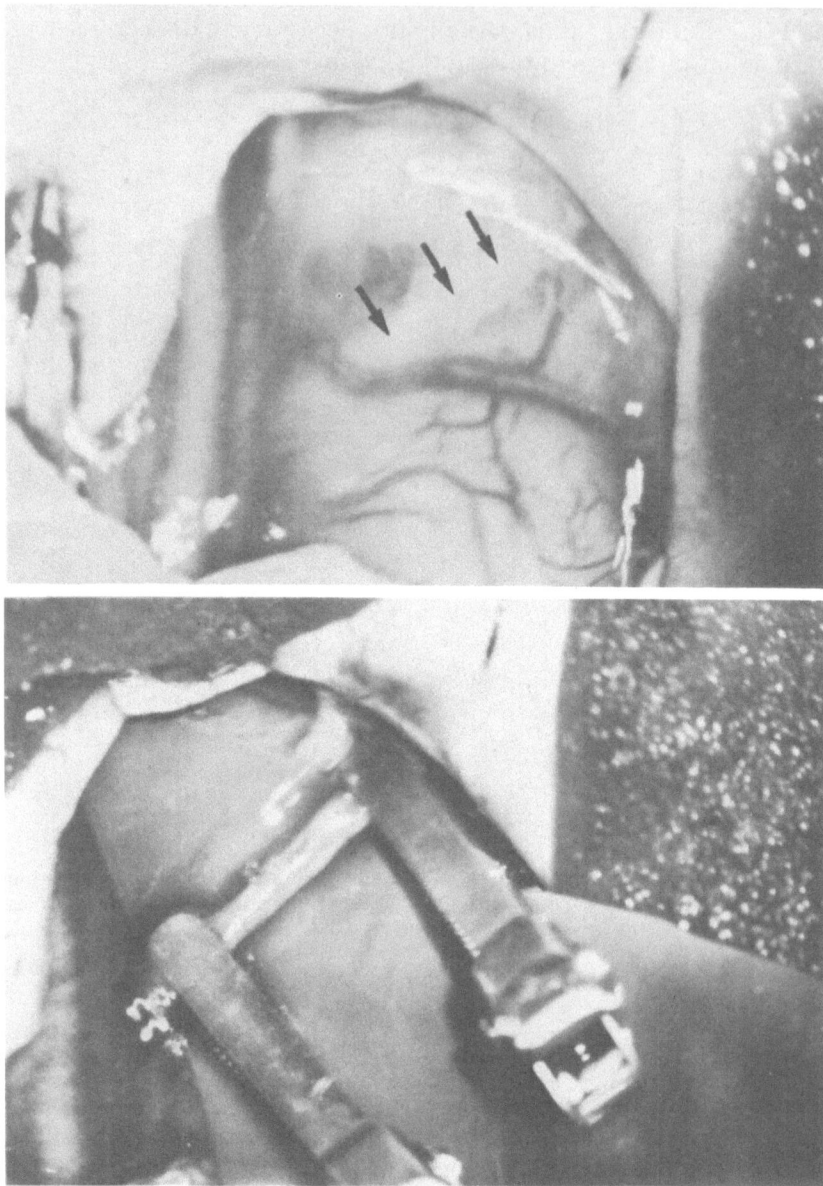

Fig. 55. An appropriate cortical vessel must be located after the burr hole has been enlarged
and the dura opened. This is often difficult in patients with a completed stroke, because the
cortical vessel is very thin due to the reduced blood supply and is often surrounded by a
thickened arachnoid. The exposure is sometimes further impeded by veins of different sizes
which either accompany or cross over the vessel. These veins should be spared to the
greatest possible extent. A triangular bit of rubber should be placed under the vessel in
order to protect the brain after the exposure and clamping of the cortical vessel

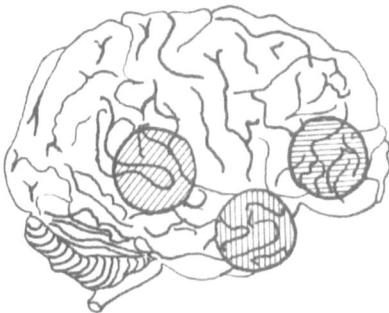

Fig. 56. A suitable cortical vessel for the anastomosis can almost certainly be found at the marked locations (according to Chater 1977)

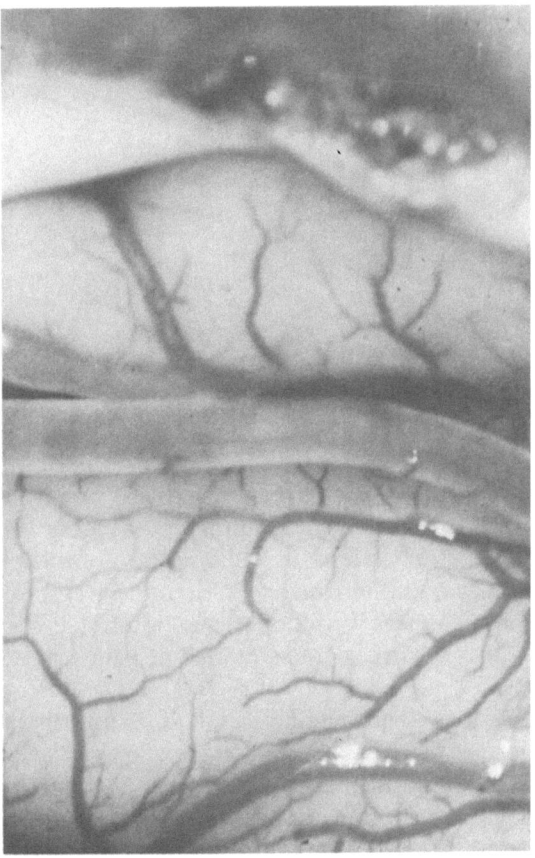

Fig. 57. An ideal cortical vessel with few collaterals

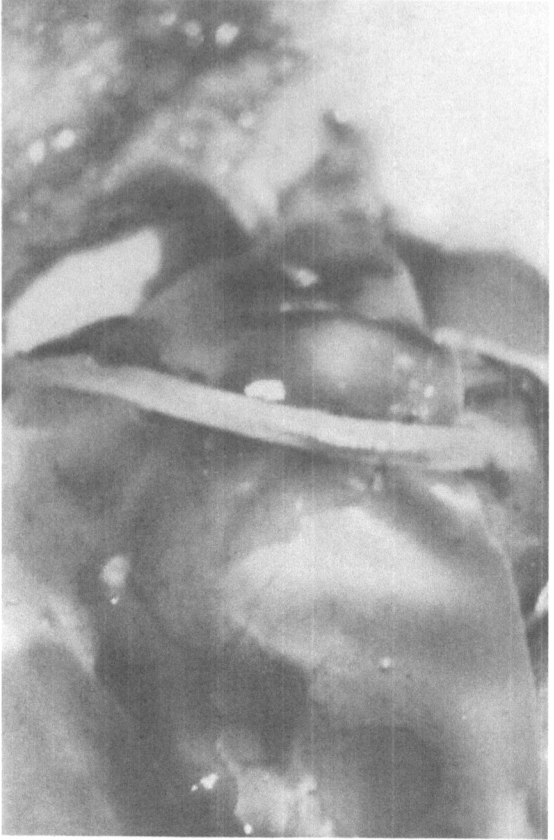

Fig. 58. A cortical vessel that was exposed a long distance

exposure some 6 cm above the external auditory meatus cortical vessels
may by found that are larger than 1 mm in diameter 100 percent of the
time. This cortical artery is part of the angular complex or the posterior
temporal complex branching from the main middle cerebral trunk. Chater
et al. feel that the success rate of 90 percent patency in 28 clinical cases in
his own material is the direct consequence of using these large recipient
arteries.

Furthermore, since a sufficiently large anastomosis has to be applied
between the microclamps, aside from the space they occupy themselves,
at least 1 cm of the vessel has to be exposed. A cortical vessel can thus be
quickly found if the burr hole is further enlarged. It is advisable to perform
a larger craniotomy rather than to use an artery of insufficient size and
thus insufficient blood supply for the anastomosis. Yonekawa and
Yaşargil (1976) suggest that the cortical vessel to be used should have a
diameter of not less than 0.8 mm and should be exposed over a section
approximately 1 cm in length.

When the cortical artery is isolated, the arachnoid around the cortical artery is opened with microscissors and the small penetrating branches to the cortex are coagulated and severed. Large bifurcating vessels can be closed temporarily with a clamp. It is absolutely necessary to check with a microdissector that there are no penetrating branches to the cortex when

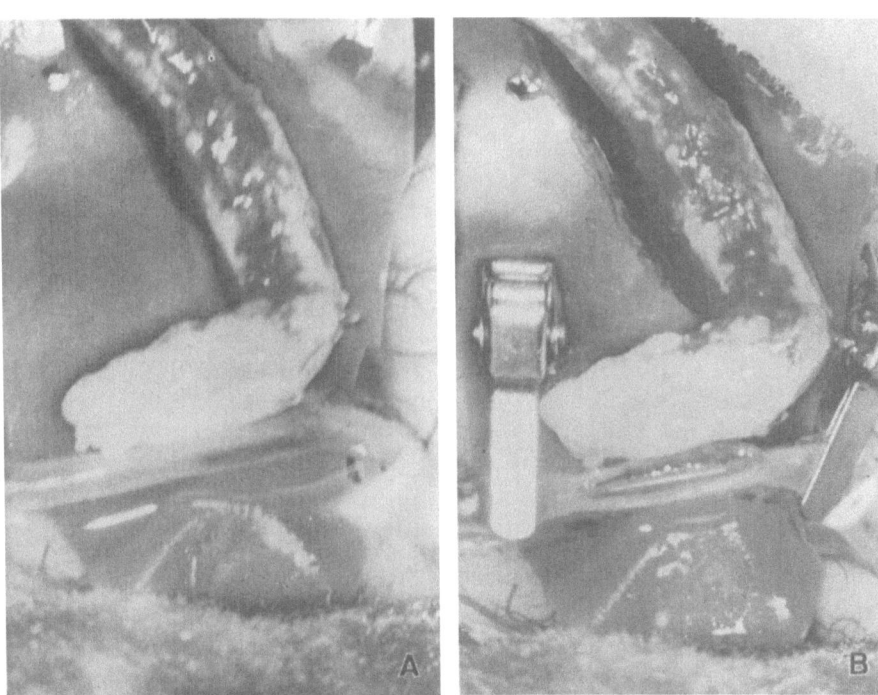

Fig. 59. Adaptation of the superficial temporal artery, preferably with a loop, to perform the anastomosis. After deciding how large the incision of the superficial temporal artery will be, the surgeon clamps cortical vessel and makes an incision of the desired length. Before the first sutures are applied, a small silicone tube may be inserted into the cortical vessel as a protective measure

the exposure is complete (Fig. 57). Such branches may cause slight but continuous hemorrhage as soon as the cortical vessel is opened to the anastomosis even after clamping. This reduces visibility and also increases considerably the risk of thrombus formation. A bit of rubber foil should be placed between the cortex and the isolated segment of the artery, both to isolate the segment and to protect the underlying cortex (Fig. 58). After the cortical vessel is completely exposed, the superficial temporal artery is clamped at its trunk and its peripheral end is dissected completely free of the surrounding connective tissue for a distance of 1.5 to 2 cm.

9.3. The Anastomosis

The end of the superficial temporal artery is now brought near the cortical vessel (Fig. 59). This enables the surgeon to determine if the superficial temporal artery is of sufficient length or if it is too long. If the vessel is not long enough, the discrepancy can be remedied by placing the skin flap closer to the burr hole. A further exposure of the superficial

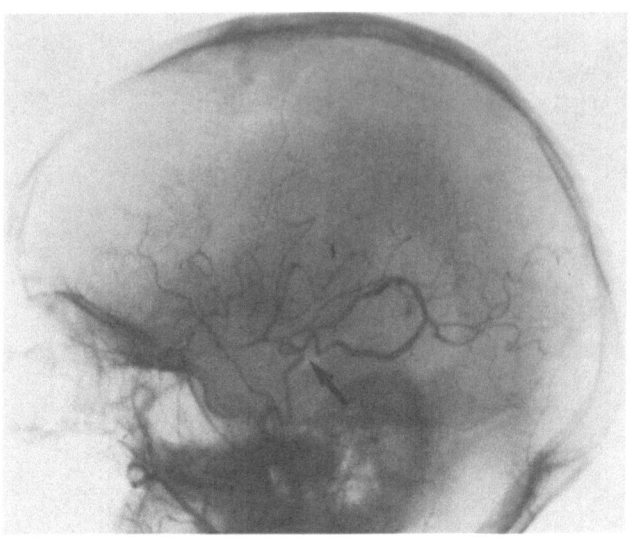

Fig. 60. A very well-functioning anastomosis with a marked dilatation of the superficial temporal artery and the cortical vessel in a 54-year-old female patient with left sided carotid occlusion. The superficial temporal artery, however, is somewhat too long. This enhances the formation of loops, which may have a negative effect on blood flow under certain conditions

temporal artery at its trunk also gains some more surface. An excessively long superficial temporal artery may cause the formation of loops (Fig. 60).

Bringing the superficial temporal artery nearer to the cortical vessel also gives the surgeon sufficient time to decide which direction the blood flow should take once the anastomosis is completed.

In their technical guidelines most authors suggest a T-shaped end-to-side anastomosis (Yaşargil 1969, Donaghy 1972, Austin 1976, Chater 1976, Gratzl et al. 1976, Yonekawa and Yaşargil 1976, Merei and Bodosi 1976) (Fig. 61). This is presumably to ensure an even distribution of blood flow to both the distal and the proximal branches of the cortical vessel (Austin 1977). On the other hand, other authors suggest that the blood flow should be directed from the superficial temporal artery toward

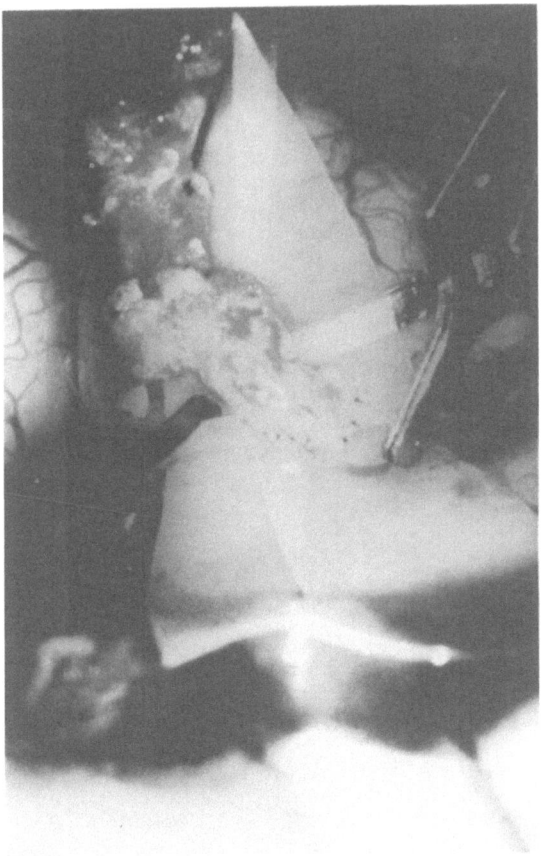

Fig. 61. A steep, T-shaped end-to-side anastomosis, with clearly visible right corner suture and sutures at the anterior wall

the sylvian fossa because large branches soon extend from the surface downward and thus provide for the irrigation of the whole middle cerebral artery region (Koos *et al.* 1976, Schuster *et al.* 1976). The anastomosis should be as wide as possible since there is always a certain tendency to shrink at the anastomosis site because of the formation of scare tissue (Chapter 6). This also enables some of the blood to reach the distal part of the vessel, even though the main blood flow is directed toward the sylvian fossa. This "patch technique" according to Koos (Fig. 62) is the basis of a satisfactory anastomosis, even when the superficial temporal artery is large and wide compared with the cortical vessel.

A longitudinal incision is then made in the superficial temporal artery on the side toward the cortical vessel and the brain. The incision must be the size of the anastomosis to be performed. The vessel must also be

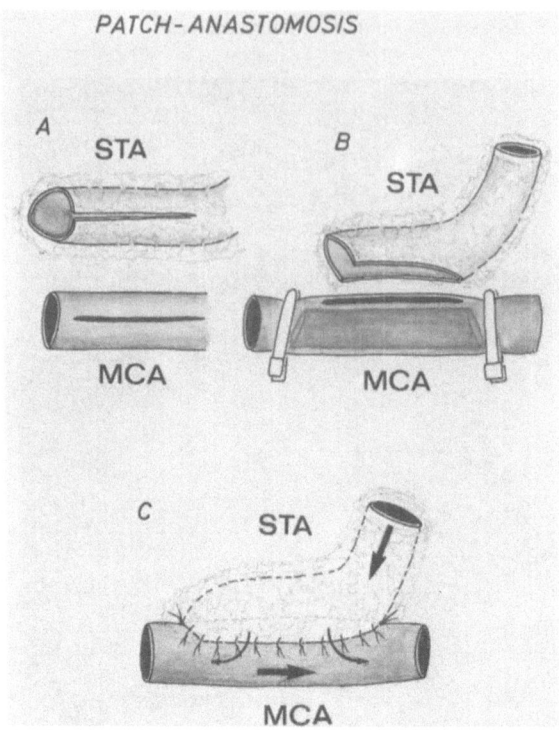

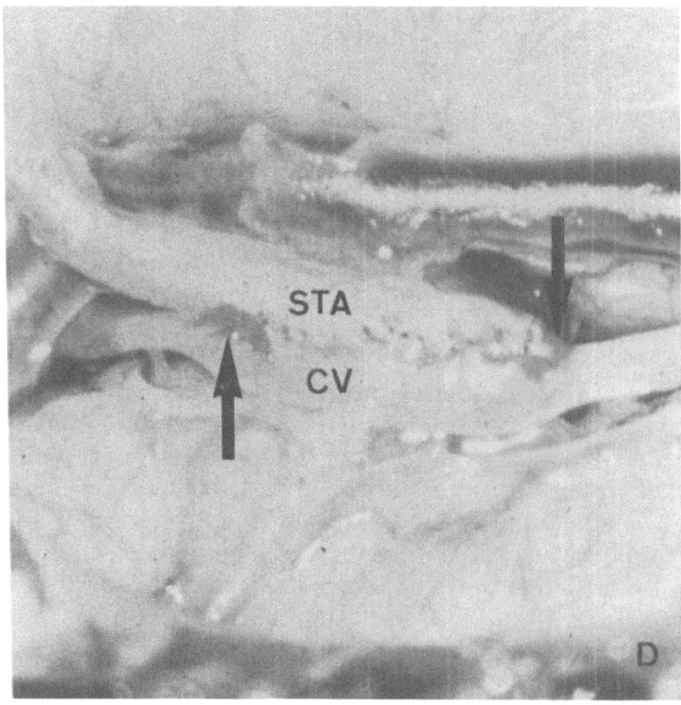

Fig. 62. A so-called "patch" anastomosis according to Koos after the clamps are opened. A very large lumen is achieved, this improves the results in regard to anastomotic function. In particular, fibrous scarring at the knots cannot lead to high-grade stenosis at a later stage. The arrows indicate the corner sutures

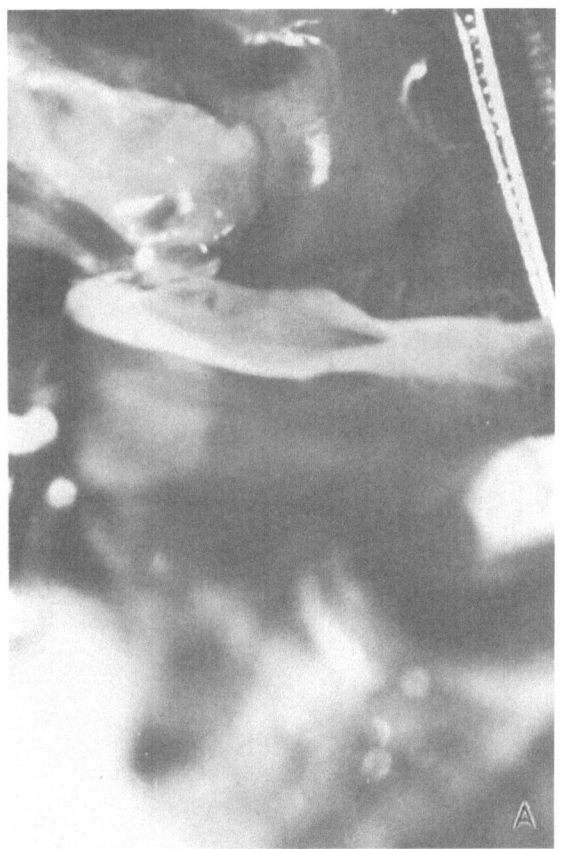

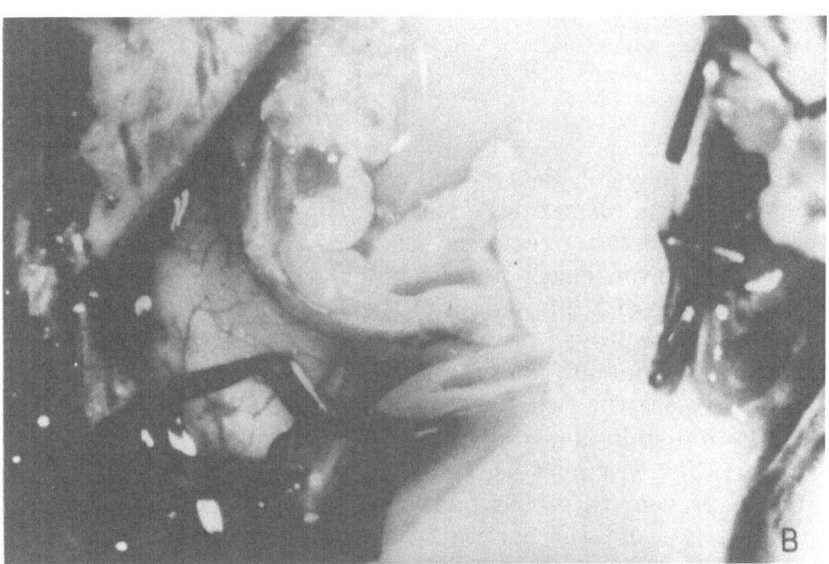

Fig. 63. The lumen of the superficial temporal artery is matched to the opened cortical vessel in order to determine the exact length before the anastomosis is sutured

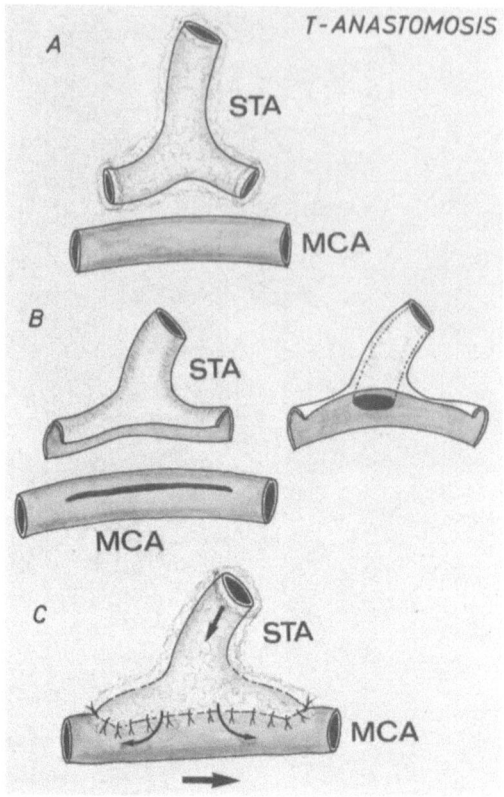

Fig. 64. T-Anastomosis using a bifurcation of the superficial temporal artery

flushed with a physiological saline solution to remove blood clots and prevent thrombus formation. After the superficial temporal artery is adapted, the cortical vessel is clamped and opened a distance corresponding to the length of incision of the superficial temporal artery (Fig. 63). The use of a bifurcation of the superficial temporal artery for anastomosis has proved to be both a very advantageous and a physiological technique. The superficial temporal artery is connected to the cortical vessel, the two vessels forming a wide T; thus blood flow is directed both distally and proximally (Fig. 64).

The cortical vessel must also be carefully flushed with a saline solution in order to prevent thrombus formation in this vessel. The superficial temporal artery and the cortical vessel are then again brought into proximity to each other. It is still possible to amend any discrepancy in the size of the incision at this stage (Fig. 63).

The corner sutures are applied first under the greatest possible magnification of the operating microscope. A good view of the opposite

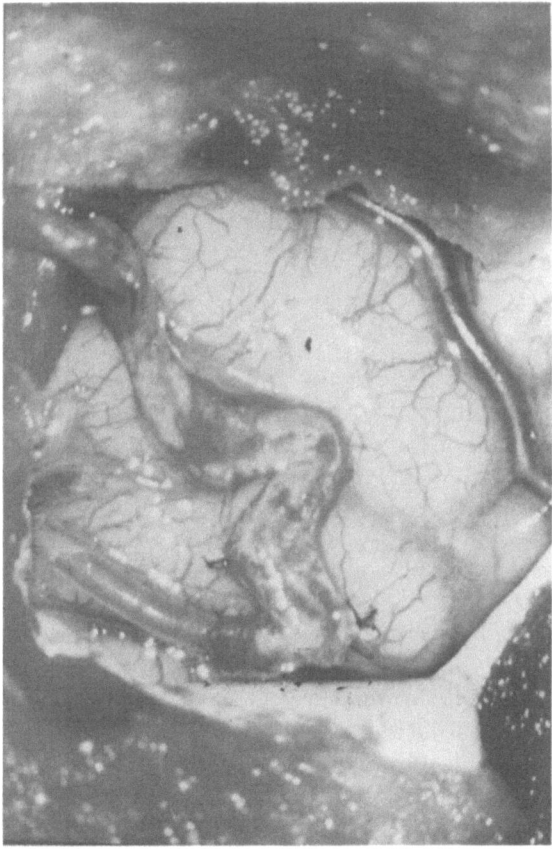

Fig. 65. After the clips are opened, good irrigation of the cortical vessel is achieved via the superficial temporal artery

wall is paramount at this stage since even a small invagination of the vascular wall may stenose or occlude the anastomosis to a considerable degree (Chapter 6).

After applying the corner sutures one should check again whether the vascular walls can now be joined without difficulty. The suturing of the anastomosis is then completed by 10-0 interrupted sutures in short regular intervals.

After completion of the suture at the posterior and anterior walls the distal clamp should be opened first, because the prevailing pressure at this site is the lowest. Under ideal conditions there is no or only slight bleeding of the anastomosis (Fig. 65). The clamp should be applied only in case of very severe bleeding. In all other instances the proximal clamp as well as the clamp at the superficial temporal artery should be opened quickly in order to restore the blood circulation. Slight or medium-grade hemorrhage from the anastomosis can be abated very quickly if conservative procedures are employed. Repeated clamping of the microanastomosis can cause

    1. another vascular lesion at the site where the clamp is placed,

    2. a risk of thrombus formation due to the stasis of the blood flow.

In many cases, an oversuturing of the bleeding site, causes a stenosis of the microanastomotic lumen (Chapter 6).

When the bleeding has stopped completely the wound must be sutured layer by layer. The dural lesion is covered by special Spongostan and Surgicel.

9.4. Intraoperative Diagnostic Procedures

The objective of intraoperative diagnostic procedures is to enable reliable identification of the ischemic region involved. A further objective is the assessment of the functional performance of the sutured microanastomosis.

Angiography, rCBF measurements, scintigraphy, and computerized tomography provide findings prior to the operation in the ischemic region. Merei (1974, 1976) uses *fluorescein angiography* for this purpose. This technique consists of intraoperative probing of the internal carotid artery with a catheter and then injection of fluorescein before exposure of the cortical vessel. The well-supplied areas are clearly visible under ultraviolet light, whereas areas with low perfusion show little or no fluorescence. This method can be used after completion of the anastomosis and also after reopening of the clamp in order to check the patency of the anastomosis. Stenoses and large lesions in the vessels required in the preceding operation can then be seen with ultraviolet light. The functional performance of the anastomosis can thus be evaluated immediately after the operation.

Another method was reported by Austin in 1974. He used Evans blue to check the patency of the anastomosis with collateral vessels via the superficial temporal artery. Ito (1976) reported on *rCBF measurement combined with intraoperative measurement of evoked potentials* (SEP). By this means he was able to detect an increase in CBF intraoperatively after the extra-intracranial anastomosis had been performed.

Spetzler (1976) mentions that *intraoperative blood flow measurements* are also valuable for determining the prognosis of a sutured microanastomosis.

The most comprehensive intraoperative studies were carried out by Yaşargil in 1974, by Chater in 1975, and by Yonekawa and Yaşargil in 1976. They consist of *intraoperative measurement of the intraluminar pressure* both in the superficial temporal artery and in the middle cerebral artery. This method allows precise determination of the difference in pressure between these two vessels, an indication of the expected anastomotic functioning. In certain cases, another cortical vessel was selected if the pressure gradient was found to be too low. This method, as well as fluorescein angiography, helps to select intraoperatively the area best suited for anastomosis.

The importance of intraoperative examinations is based on the fact that to a certain extent the functional activity of the microanastomosis can be evaluated at operation. If these findings correlate with preoperative tests—particularly rCBF measurements and computerized tomography—the information provided by such preoperative examinations could become more and more precise in the future.

9.5. Intra- and Postoperative Complications

From a technical point of view, an extra-intracranial anastomosis is not a particularly risky operation. It is performed essentially in the scalp region and at the surface of the brain. Regardless of the apparent easiness of the operation it should be kept in mind that under certain circumstances considerable changes in blood flow and changes in intracranial arterial circulation may take place. These may lead to repercussions affecting even the area supplied by the extracranial vessels (Chapter 13).

Spasms of the cortical vessels, which can severely affect the functional performance of the anastomosis during the operation are of major importance. Spasms are particularly noticed whenever the cortical vessels are not handled carefully; this means that the occurrence of a spasm depends directly on the surgical technique of the operation. The spasm of the cortical vessels usually disappears spontaneously after 10 minutes. If it does not disappear, administration of papaverin is advisable (Yaşargil 1969, Yonekawa and Yaşargil 1976).

Another striking effect although not an immediate complication, is the substantial *increase in blood pressure* that is usually noted after reopening all the clamps. Sometimes, this increase is so high that it affects the patient's condition seriously and jeopardizes the successful outcome of the operation.

Blood pressure has to be monitored very carefully after the clamps are opened. This observation was also made by Yaşargil (1970), Austin (1975), Gratzl (1975), Reichmann (1975), and Yonekawa (1976). The increased blood pressure can be explained by the excessive perfusion of a previously ischemic region. The ischemic area requires an increase of blood flow and volume; this obviously causes an increase in systemic blood pressure.

In a 57-year-old patient with a preoperative blood pressure of 180 mm Hg, after completion of the extra-intracranial anastomosis and after all the clamps were opened, blood pressure rose to more than 240 mm Hg. Immediately after the operation, the patient suffered a stroke located contralaterally to the anastomosis (Case 35).

A further complication occasionally mentioned is the occurrence of *seizures*. Yonekawa and Yaşargil (1976) reported seizures in 3 to 10 percents of patients, and Reichmann (1976) in 5 from 80 patients. At the Department of Neurosurgery, Vienna, seizures were observed immediately following the operation in only 2 of 100 patients operated upon.

The most serious complications noticed were *occlusions and stenoses of the intracranial vessels* or the afferent cerebral arteries shortly after operation. Such complications seem to be caused by steal phenomena, although their cause has not been completely clarified as yet (Kletter 1978; see also Chapter 13).

Another complication may be postoperative deterioration in the neurological condition for a few days, caused mainly by an intracerebral or *intracranial steal phenomenon* (Kletter 1978).

No waterproof closure can be performed where the superficial temporal artery penetrates the bone and the dura toward the cortex. Thus

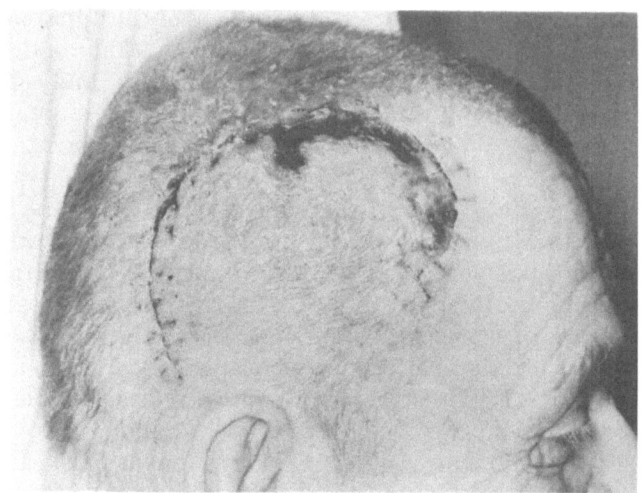

Fig. 66. Scalp flap necrosis 20 days after extra-intracranial bypass operation

a *spinalfluid cushion* is invariably found postoperatively above the site of the craniotomy. It usually disappears spontaneously within 1 week. This absorption process can be accelerated by puncturing the cushion (Yonekawa and Yaşargil 1975, Reichmann 1976).

Scalp flap necrosis may often occur because the superficial temporal artery supplies the skin flap. Conservative treatment is usually sufficient and in most cases plastic surgery is not necessary (Reichmann 1976, Chater 1977) (Fig. 66). Direct exposure of the superficial temporal artery without a skin flap can prevent this complication.

A postoperative *subdural hematoma* has sometimes been observed after treatment with anticoagulants (Reichmann 1976).

In addition to complications occurring immediately after the operation there are a number of specific late complications such as pulmonary embolism and cardiac infarction, which are not necessarily characteristic of neurosurgery and may occur after any surgery.

Postoperative and later causes of death are discussed in Chapter 14.

10. Postoperative Examinations

The *neurological examination*, as mentioned in Chapter 7 (Preoperative Diagnostic Procedures) is the only method that can be performed reliably immediately after the operation and the only one that can detect changes in patients who exhibit a neurological deficit prior to the operation.

Palpation is a very reliable procedure for monitoring the functional activity *of the superficial temporal artery*. Since the superficial temporal artery expands immediately after surgery (provided that indication and technique were adequate), a substantially higher pulsation of this vessel is noticeable on the first postoperative day (Yaşargil 1970, Austin 1975; Yonekawa and Yaşargil 1975). However, Yaşargil (1973) reported that in some cases the pulsation of the superficial temporal artery dropped considerably on the second, third, and fourth postoperative days. This was a result of the postoperative histological changes (dealt with in Chapter 6). Increased thrombus formation in the microanastomotic region is the cause of the reduction of blood flow. The reduced flow is reflected in the reduced pulsation of the superficial temporal artery. If the pulsation of this vessel decreases and a complete stasis occurs after 5 days, one may assume that the microanastomosis is occluded. Awareness of this fact is essential whenever palpation findings are unfavorable. Follow-up angiography should be performed immediately after operation in order not to lose time in determining if another operation or extra-intracranial anastomosis is required. If the functioning of the anastomosis is satisfactory, however, the pulsation of the superficial temporal artery will increase again on the fifth day and will rise continuously.

The *four-vessel angiography* is the most important postoperative examination method after the neurological examination. It reveals
1. the function of the anastomosis,
2. the size of the supplied area,
3. any changes in the collateral circulation.

For many years, the timing of the angiography postoperatively has been rather controversial. Premature angiography was believed to cause vascular spasms and various changes in the region of the anastomosis (Yaşargil 1969; Reichmann 1972; Yonekawa and Yaşargil 1976). In recent years angiography has usually been performed before the patient is discharged from the hospital, approximately 7 to 10 days after the operation (Merei 1973, Gratzl 1976). It is true that if performed too early, angiography fails to show the full extent of dilatation of the superficial temporal artery and its supplied area. However, conclusions about the anastomotic function can be drawn even if the diameter is only slightly enlarged. Later angiographies, which can be performed after an early follow-up angiography, reveal a further enlargement of the lumen and the area supplied (Reichmann 1970, Chater 1976, Deruty *et al.* 1976, Gratzl *et al.* 1976). In particular, it can then be observed whether or not the anastomosis functions. If the anastomosis is occluded, the operation should either be revised or a new bypass should be performed with another

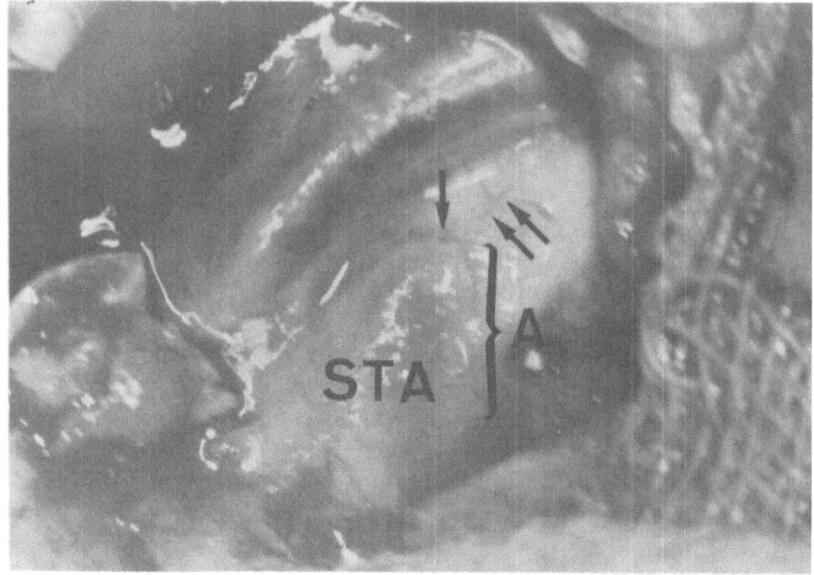

Fig. 67. A thrombosed extra-intracranial anastomosis 10 days after the operation. A large thrombus fills the lumen of the superficial temporal artery (*STA*). The cortical vessel is bloodless (arrows). The upper corner suture is clearly visible (arrow)

vessel, for example, the occipital artery. It is desirable to perform an angiography on every patient about 1 week after operation as well as six months later. This is often rather difficult, since many patients are unwilling to undergo additional angiography, especially if their postoperative status has greatly improved. This it is the reason that only 40 to 60 percent of all bypass patients submit themselves to postoperative angiography. Regardless of the fact that the angiogram is of greater importance at a later stage, angiography should be performed while the

Fig. 68. A) Due to an occluded anastomosis (see Fig. 67), the occipital artery is exposed over a length of 15 cm. B) After the previous incision has been reopend, the occipital artery (white arrow) is passed underneath the skin flap toward the opening used in the previous craniotomy (arrows). C) The anastomosis between the occipital artery (*OA*) and the cortical vessel (*CV*) is sutured

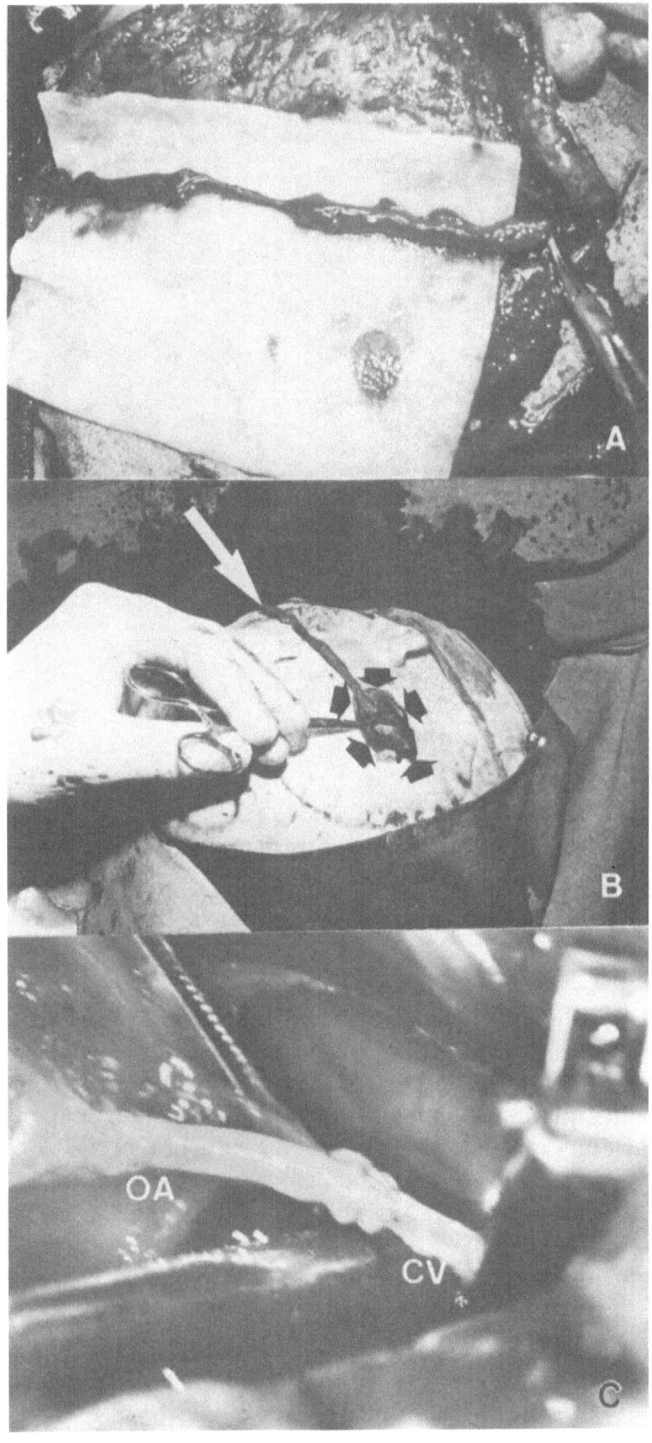

Fig. 68

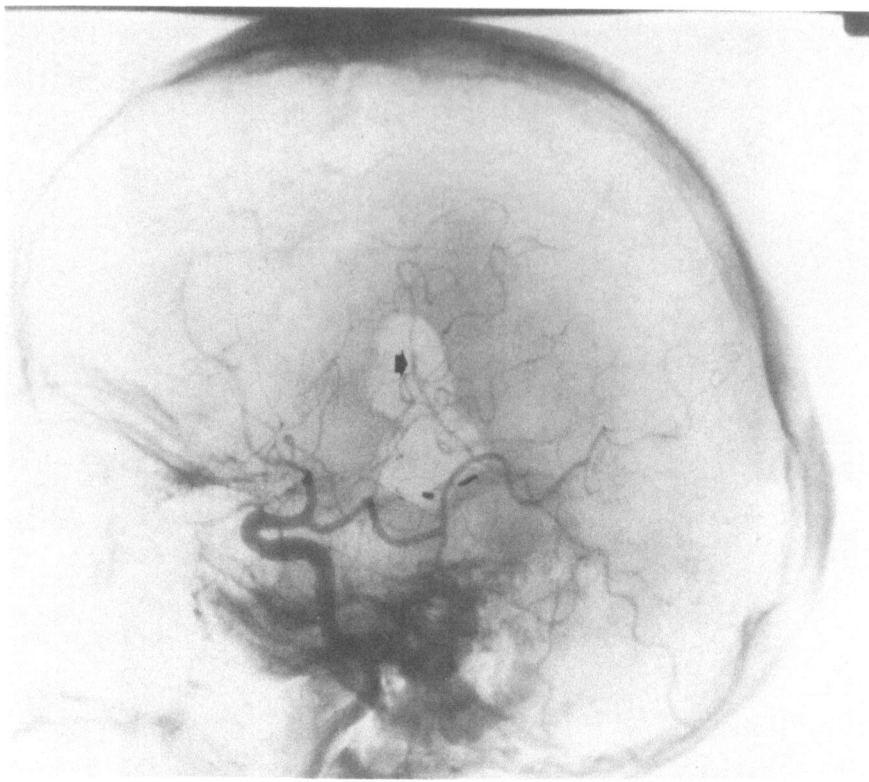

Fig. 69. A medium-grade dilatation of the occipital artery 3 weeks postoperatively with a good functioning anastomosis (arrow) and satisfactory perfusion of the region of the middle cerebral artery. Caudal to the anastomosis, there is a small poorly vascularized area, which corresponds approximately to the thrombosed first anastomosis and the thrombosed cortical vessel

patient is still in hospital, especially if it is indicated—for example, if a subdural hematoma or an intracerebral hemorrhage is suspected.

Angiography can also be performed at any time after the operation without causing adverse effects on the patient or jeopardizing the results of the operation. For these reasons one should not hesitate to perform angiography even a few hours after the extra-intracranial bypass if it appears to be necessary or advisable; thus no precious time is lost if further action is required.

If an occlusion of the anastomosis has been verified by postoperative angiography, an attempt may be made to revise the operation. The vessels in the anastomosis region are usually occluded by large thrombi, which then may require thrombectomy (Fig. 67). Thrombectomy is often easier to perform in the region of the superficial temporal artery than in the region of the cortical vessel because the wall of the latter is very brittle. The manipulations required in thrombectomy can cause massive endothelial lesions and thus make the formation of new thrombi quite probable. In such cases, it is preferable to use the ipsilateral occipital artery for a new bypass (Kletter 1978).

Figure 67 shows the anastomosis of a 57-year-old patient with embolic middle cerebral artery occlusion. The extra-intracranial bypass was occluded 1 week after the operation. Ten days after the first operation, the occipital artery was used for another extra-intracranial bypass, performed at a distance of about 1 cm from the previous anastomosis (Fig. 68). The patient's neurological condition was unchanged prior to the second operation. After the occipital bypass, his condition improved in a few days after operation (Fig. 69).

The use of *Doppler sonography*, *EEG*, and *scintigraphy* for monitoring postoperative improvement of the patient's general condition is of limited value. The echograms do not exhibit different readings after the operation, particularly after a carotid occlusion. However, the functional performance of the bypass can be detected very well by Doppler sonography at any time without strain to the patient. Regular check-ups by means of this method are very feasible and can provide valuable data about the anastomotic function through changes in pulsation of the superficial temporal artery.

EEG can reveal improvement in blood flow, usually somewhat later after surgery. The EEG is essential in detecting postoperative seizures, which occur occasionally (Reichmann 1974).

Only a few neurosurgical centers take rCBF measurements both before and after an operation as well as later postoperatively (Austin 1973; Heilbrunn 1974; Gratzl et al. 1975; Ito 1976; Schmiedek et al. 1977). Such measurements have proven that rCBF can improve substantially under favorable conditions such as correct indication and proper surgical technique. Schmiedek et al. (1977) performed rCBF studies in 33 cases both pre- and postoperatively. In 10 patients, CBF measurements were again performed about 1 year after the operation. In 4 of these patients CBF measurements revealed a substantial improvement and a high increase in blood flow as compared to preoperative measurements. In 2 patients, a particularly good increase in blood flow was observed.

rCBF measurement is the best method for obtaining detailed findings about the extent of local blood flow improvement postoperatively (Fig. 70). Since a visible increase in rCBF is always associated with satisfactory function of the anastomosis and improvement in neurological condition, postoperative verification does not usually require routine rCBF measurement. This evidence is provided by angiography and clinical improvement of the patient's condition. Clinical improvement can only occur if sufficient brain tissue recovers after reconstructive surgery. In the case of a well-functioning anastomosis but insufficient neurological recovery, rCBF measurement does not improve postoperatively (Schmiedek et al. 1976). In an occluded anastomosis, rCBF is either unchanged or later even substantially reduced; this is a further sign of brain degeneration.

rCBF measurement thus does not necessarily have to be performed after the operation. Schmiedek *et al.* 1976, who carried out the most comprehensive pre- and postoperative studies also concluded "that this method is not particularly suited for routine examinations pre- and postoperatively".

The use of this method, however, has contributed in a decisive way to demonstrating that the extra-intracranial bypass yields satisfactory results and that its application is to be recommended.

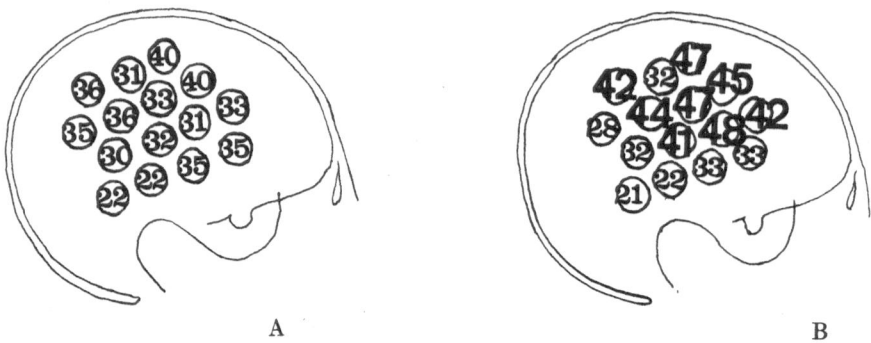

A   B

Fig. 70. Postoperative measurement (B) of rCBF provides objective data in regard to the function of the anastomosis and the present blood supply to the brain region above the anastomosis that showed low-perfusion preoperatively (A) (according to Schmiedek and Gratzl 1977)

The use of *postoperative computerized tomography* following extra-intracranial bypass is too recent to allow a definite evaluation. First results show, however, that this method can also reveal an improved blood flow whenever increased density is visible in the damaged area (Chater *et al.* 1978; Reisner *et al.* 1978).

10.1. Conclusion

The most essential postoperative examination methods are neurological tests and neuropsychiatric examinations. These provide the best basis for evaluating the patient's actual postoperative condition. Four-vessel angiography is best suited to evaluation of the anastomotic function, the size of the supplied area, and any changes that occur in collateral circulation (Chapter 13). All the other postoperative examinations are not absolutely necessary to demonstrate the satisfactory functioning of the anastomosis and improvement of the patient's condition. The computerized tomography is not necessary but can provide good data of improved or unchanged blood flow.

In specific cases, however, they are certainly advisable—for example, if it is necessary to trace epileptic potentials by EEG or to demonstrate the extent of rCBF improvement by making these measurements.

11. Indications for Extra-Intracranial Bypass Procedure: Pathological-Anatomical Considerations

Pathological changes alone are not a sufficient indication for an extra-intracranial bypass operation. Pathological changes must always be considered in relation to the clinically symptoms. Thus if the patient does not have any TIA in his case history nor any neurological symptoms, and if scintigraphy, CBF measurements, and computerized tomography do not reveal any pathological findings, surgery is not indicated, although the patient may have, for example, an occlusion of the internal carotid artery. Extra-intracranial anastomosis is also definitely contraindicated in cases in which neurological deficits are not accompanied by pathological anatomical changes. Such patients, however, must be carefully monitored and re-examined at regular intervals. They should be instructed to report immediately sudden deterioration in their visual acuity, dizziness, or increasing headaches, so that new tests can be performed. Routine check-ups can be helpful in detecting disorders that the patient himself is unaware of. Reduced mental activity in particular is often noticed as the first stage of a clinically manifest occlusion. In any case, it should be remembered that progressive arteriosclerosis in patients with vascular lesions can gradually affect existing collateral circulation, which may then cause a stenosis or even an occlusion in these regions.

Regardless of the morphological changes, an additional angiography of the lesioned vessel part should be made immediately before the operation. Spontaneous recanalization occurs quite often, and vascular spasms are sometimes mistaken for stenoses (Figs. 37, 38, pages 47, 48).

11.1. Occlusion of the Internal Carotid Artery

11.1.1. Extracranial Portion

Extracranial occlusions of the internal carotid artery usually can not be cervically eliminated because of the missing link with the periphery. This condition is ideal for an extra-intracranial bypass operation from a morphological point of view because it is often associated with only slight neurological deficits. This is the reason that operations on carotid occlusions are statistically in the highest percentage (Table 6, page 101). Figures 71 A, B, and 72 A, B show an carotid occlusion in a 55-year-old female patient with slight hemiparesis on the right side and a high-grade aphasia. Four weeks after the operation, the paresis had receded and only moderate aphasia was still present. This symptom also disappeared almost completely within 6 months.

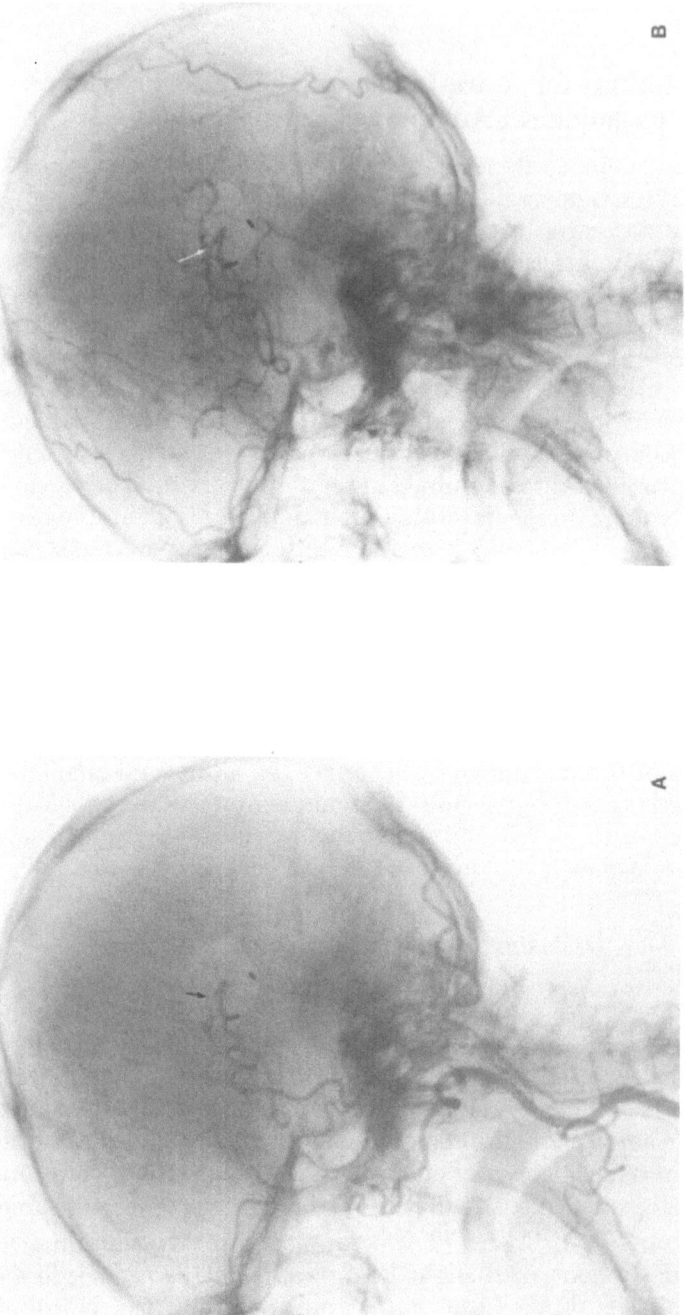

Fig. 71. A 55-year-old femal patient (case 30) with left sided carotid occlusion, high-grade hemiparesis on the right, and motor aphasia 8 weeks before the operation. A) The angiogram made 9 days postoperatively shows a slightly dilated superficial temporal artery (difference between the parietal and the frontal branch), with initial supply to the cortical vessel. B) The late phase of the angiogram shows a very good supply to the region of the middle cerebral artery through the anastomosis (arrow)

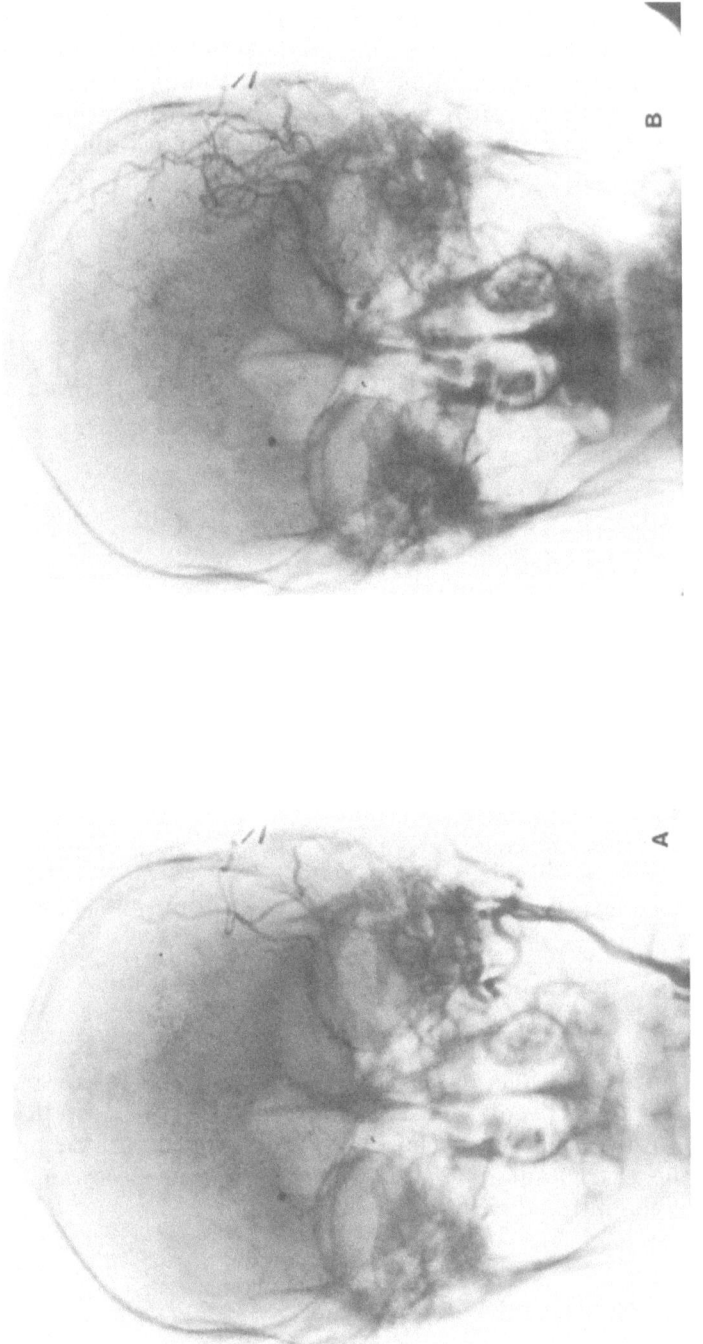

Fig. 72. Anteroposterior projection of the case shown in Fig. 71

At present, acute occlusions of the internal carotid artery cannot be treated surgically. Although surgery on acute carotid occlusions have sometimes been reported as being successful, in most cases it has been unfavorable and thus surgery seems inadvisable at an acute stage of occlusion. If an operation is intended at all, an attempt should be made to approach the acute carotid occlusion by the direct cervical method because a satisfactory connection can then usually be established distally.

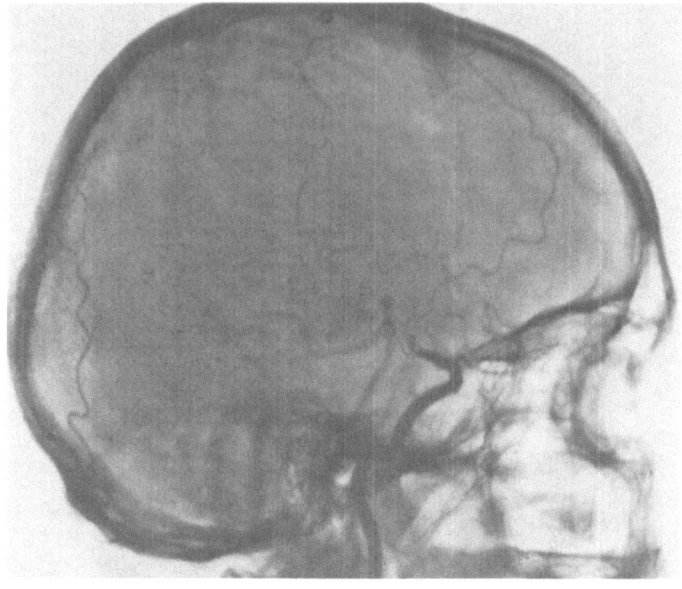

Fig. 73. Carotid occlusion in the intracranial region in a 65-year-old patient

11.1.2. Intracranial Portion

Intracranial occlusions of the internal carotid artery are also ideal indications for an extra-intracranial bypass (Fig. 73). Such conditions are quite rare, however, since an occlusion of the internal carotid artery tends to affect the extracranial portion which then appear as an cervical occlusion of the internal carotid artery.

11.2. Stenoses of the Internal Carotid Artery

Stenoses in the extracranial portion of the internal carotid artery should be approached directly whenever possible. If the stenosis cannot be reached cervically or if it is located in the intracranial portion, an extra-

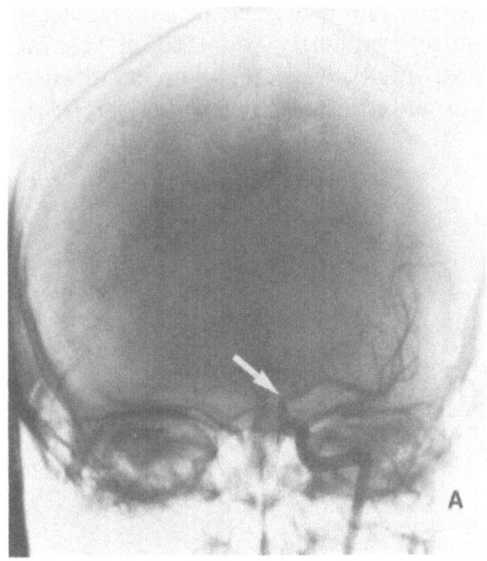

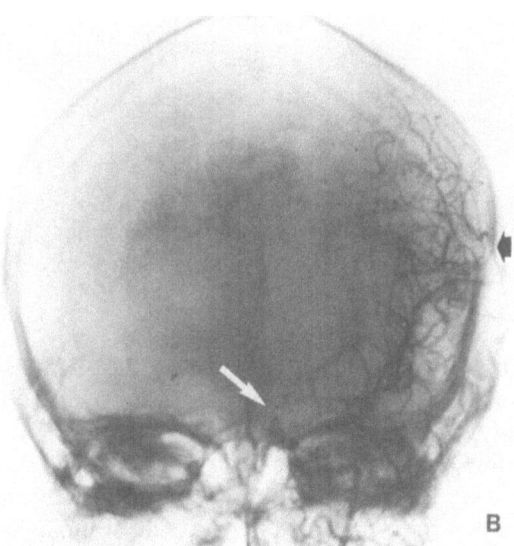

Fig. 74. A 34-year-old female patient with high-grade stenosis of the internal carotid artery in the intracranial region (case 3). Postoperatively, there is very good postoperative perfusion of the middle cerebral artery region via the anastomosis. The stenosis in the intracranial region has developed into an occlusion (B)

intracranial operation should be performed. Hemodynamic factors can account for changes in the blood flow which may then cause an occlusion of the existing stenosis. This occurred in several cases included in our study. Cases are quite frequently reported in the literature in which difficulties arose postoperatively and even resulted in fatalities after operations on siphon stenoses or intracranial stenoses (Yaşargil 1972,

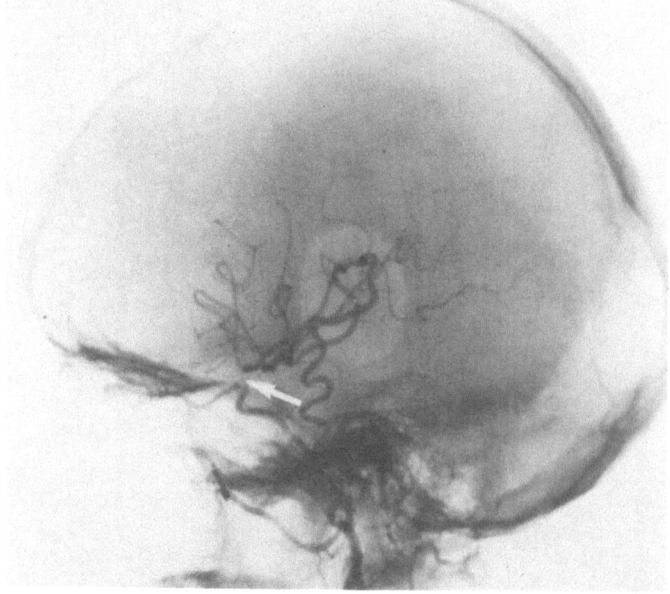

Fig. 75. Lateral postoperative angiogram of patient shown in Fig. 74. There is very good dilatation of the superficial temporal artery with good blood supply to the middle cerebral artery region, and occlusion of the internal carotid artery in the intracranial part (↑)

Chater 1976). This problem is dealt with in depth in Chapter 13. The following two factors must be taken into account in these types of lesions:
1. degree of stenosis,
2. degree of neurological deficit.
If a high-grade stenosis in the siphon part of the internal carotid artery exists, then there is a high probability that the stenosis will develop into an occlusion shortly after the operation (Figs. 74 and 75). Even if the stenosis is not too severe and surgery appears to be indicated, there is still the risk that hemodynamic factors will cause the stenosis to develop into an occlusion within a short period of time. In extra-intracranial anastomosis performed on stenoses in the carotid siphon or in the intracranial portion of the internal carotid artery, one should always consider whether the neurological deficits caused by postoperative

occlusion of the stenosis or an insufficient anastomosis would not be more severe postoperatively than preoperatively. One should keep in mind that a stenosis in this area can spontaneously turn into an occlusion within a short period of time (Chapter 13).

This process usually takes longer if it is not provoked by blood flow and pressure changes induced by surgery.

Figure 74 shows the left-sided angiogram of a 34-year-old female with slight hemiparesis on the right side. In the intracranial portion of the carotid artery there was a high-grade stenosis. One week after the operation the stenosis was changed into an occlusion (Figs. 74 B, 75, see also Figs. 93 and 94). The extra-intracranial bypass supplied the region of the middle cerebral artery. Two weeks after operation the patient had no neurological deficit.

11.3. Occlusion of the Middle Cerebral Artery

The occlusion of the middle cerebral artery is sometimes an embolic process. Such an occlusion is frequently accompanied by severe neurological deficit, so that on the basis of the clinical findings alone reconstructive vascular surgery seems inadvisable. It is surprising, however, that neurological symptoms sometimes improve substantially following an extra-intracranial bypass, even if there had been severe neurological deficits. Preoperative scintigraphy, rCBF measurements and computerized tomography can best indicate the following; whether or not surgery is recommended, the amount of depleted brain tissue, and whether or not a neurological improvement can be expected to follow. The operation should be performed not later than 8 weeks after the appearance of the occlusion because of the likelihood of an increasing decay of the cells that have already reached the limits of decompensation (Chapter 12.3.).

Thus high-grade lesions associated with large malacic cysts can be seen by means of computerized tomography as early as 4 weeks after their appearance. Surgery is not indicated in such cases (Fig. 76).

In the author's opinion the best time for an operation following infarction is 5 to 8 weeks after the attack (Table 4, page 60) (Fig. 77 and Fig. 78 A, B).

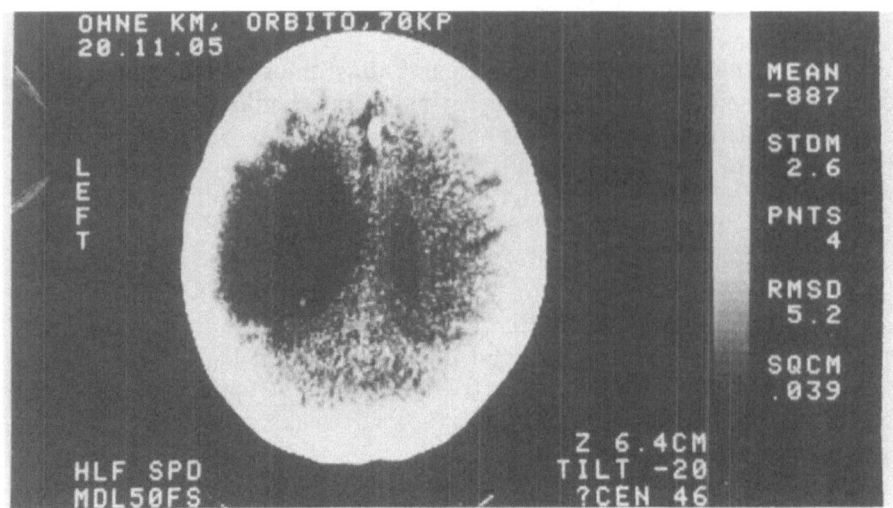

Fig. 76. Computerized tomogram of a 73-year-old patient with a left sided middle cerebral artery occlusion and a cyst in the occluded region. Surgery is contraindicated

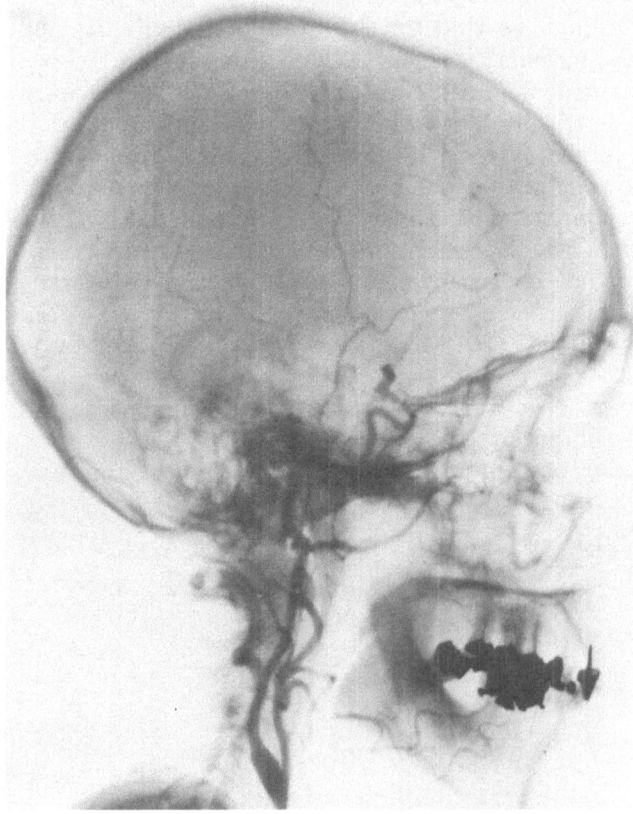

Fig. 77. A 46-year-old female patient (case 36) with embolic occlusion of the middle cerebral artery at its bifurcation from the internal carotid artery

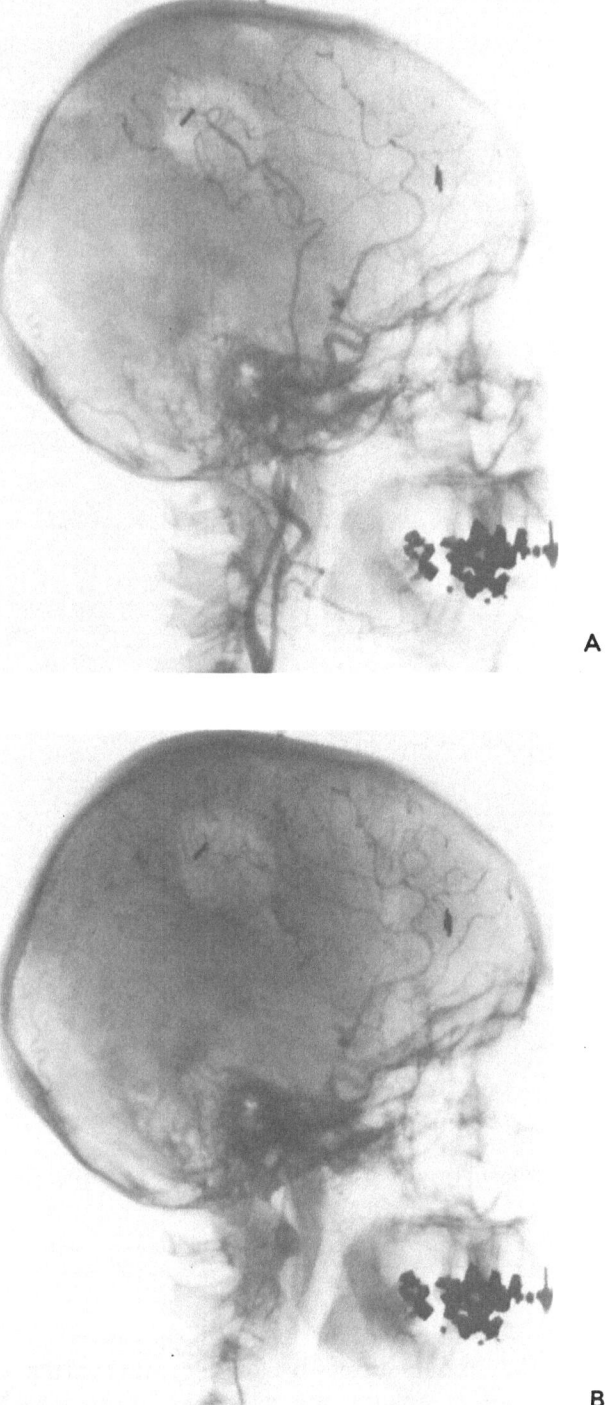

A

B

Fig. 78. Angiogram of patient shown in Fig. 77 made 8 days postoperatively reveals a marked-dilatation of the parietal branch of the superficial temporal artery, that was used in the operation. The frontal branch has a much smaller diameter than in the preoperative angiogram. A) The anastomotic function is very satisfactory. B) The whole MCA region is well supplied by the anastomosis

11.4. Stenosis of the Middle Cerebral Artery

Stenosis in the region of the middle cerebral artery is a rather controversial indication for extra-intracranial bypass. First, one should bear in mind that spasms following slight hemorrhages are occasionally mistaken for stenoses in the MCA region. Second,

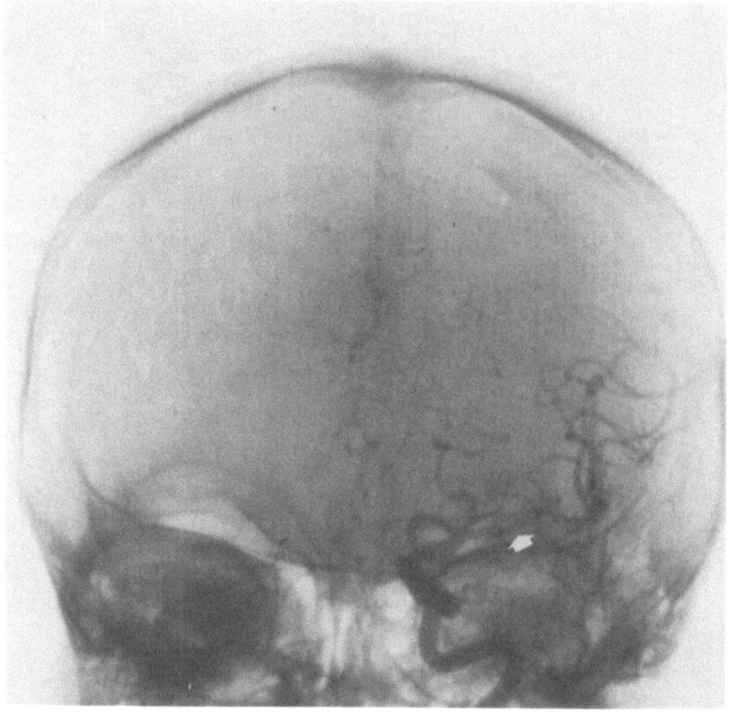

Fig. 79. High-grade middle cerebral artery stenosis in a 63-year-old patient (case 27) with hemiparesis on the right side

clinically manifest stenoses of the middle cerebral artery region have been to be undetectable by angiography after several weeks. Spasms in the acute phase, recanalization and shrinkage of small clots are difficult to differentiate from one another. If the stenosis of the vessel section is patent again after the operation, the extra-intracranial anastomosis may be altogether useless. Hemodynamic factors may also cause occlusion or insufficiency of the anastomosis.

Austin (1977) expressed the opinion that surgery should not be

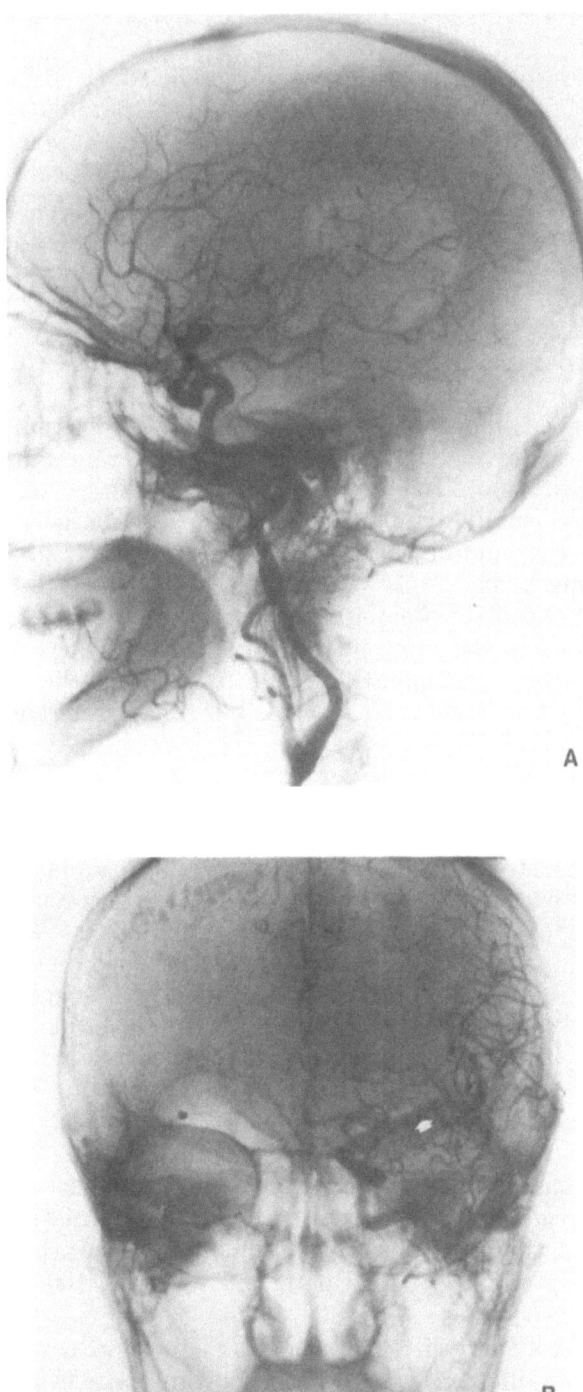

Fig. 80. A) Angiogram 4 weeks after of patient shown in Fig. 79 shows no dilatation of the superficial temporal artery. The anastomosis is hardly visible. This is due to the recanalization of the preoperative middle cerebral artery stenosis (B)

performed unless blood flow is significantly reduced. If CBF measurement reveals a blood flow reduction of over 25 percent, the slightest decrease in blood pressure may result in an attack. In this case, surgery is indicated although no symptoms are manifest as yet. Patients who are not operated upon because the CBF is not substantially lowered must be monitored and re-examined periodically.

The anastomotic function may be unsatisfactory if no massive stenosis exists and the anastomosis may occlude later because of the insufficient pressure gradient. This phenomenon has been reported by various authors (Yonekawa and Yaşargil 1975, case 5, Schmiedek et al. 1976, Gratzl et al. 1976).

Cases have been reported in which the blood flow passing through the anastomosis was reversed, flowing in an extracranial instead of an intracranial direction. In any case, only stenoses of the middle cerebral artery main trunk are suitable for surgery. Peripheral occlusions of the middle cerebral artery can be treated best with conservative methods.

Figure 79 A shows the preoperative angiogram of a 63-years-old female with hemiparesis on the right side and a stenosis of the middle cerebral artery. Four weeks postoperatively the function of the bypass is not clearly visible. The angiogram revealed recanalization of the middle cerebral artery (Figs. 80 A, B).

11.5. Occlusions and Stenoses in the Vertebrobasilar Region

In cases of isolated changes in this region, a direct anastomosis can be performed, for example, between the occipital artery and the posterior inferior artery of the cerebellum (Khodadad 1976, Weinstein 1978). Sclerotic and degenerative vascular changes in the region of the posterior cranial fossa are usually found only together with severe pathological changes. Yonekawa and Yaşargil (1976) do not mention any vertebro-basilar lesions in 65 patients on whom extra-intracranial anastomosis was performed. Stephens (1977) describes 10 patients with an extra-intracranial bypass, 3 of whom also had a stenosis or occlusion in a vertebral artery. Gratzl et al. (1976) describe about 65 cases of extra-intracranial anastomosis without mentioning changes in the vessels located in the region of the posterior cranial fossa. Deruty (1974) does not specifically mention any vertebrobasilar lesions in the 15 patients included in his study, nor does Chater (1976) in the 100 patients in his study.

There is hardly any literature on this subject. Because the severe lesions, which are incidently of major importance, are caused mainly by changes in the carotid region, and isolated vertebrobasilar lesions are extremely rare. Extra-intracranial anastomosis via the middle cerebral artery can also influence the vertebrobasilar area (Khodadad 1976, Weinstein 1978). One must, however, consider the fact that patients with acute basilar occlusions have a very high mortality rate.

11.6. Multiple Vascular Lesions

Because arteriosclerosis affects the entire vascular system, it is not at all surprising that in many patients on whom extra-intracranial anastomosis was performed, not only one, but several vessels were occluded. Patients with multiple vascular stenoses or occlusions run a significantly higher risk of having a stroke or dying of acute apoplexy. It is for this reason that an extra-intracranial bypass operation in cases of multiple vascular changes in intra- and extracranial regions is of particular importance. In his study, Chater (1976) observed that 28 of 100 patients had multiple lesions. Stephens (1973) detected such changes in 8 of 10 patients, and Yonekawa and Yaşargil (1976) in 24 of 65. According to Gratzl et al. (1976) 11 of 65 patients who underwent anastomosis had multiple vascular changes in the intracranial region. In our own study, 14 of 80 patients had multiple vascular changes (Table 6). It may be

Table 6. *Sites of Steno-Occlusive Lesions (n = 80)*

Bilateral internal carotid occlusion	2
Unilateral internal carotid occlusion	42
Unilateral internal carotid occlusion + Stenosis of contralateral carotid artery	12
Stenosis of Siphon	7
Occlusion of middle cerebral artery	9
Stenosis of middle cerebral artery	5
Angioma	1
Aneurysm	1
Moya-Moya	1

assumed that between 30 to 60 percent of the patients operated upon had multiple vascular changes in the intra- and extracranial regions, although many authors do not describe these multiple changes in detail. It is striking that a patient with a stenosis—for example, in the region of the internal carotid artery—may have another stenosis contralaterally, at exactly the same site (Figs. 81, 82). In such a case only the side that has manifest clinical symptoms or low CBF will be operated upon in accordance with the general guidelines pertaining to indication for extra-intracranial bypass. Most comprehensive statistical surveys on extra-intracranial anastomosis include several cases in which anastomosis was performed bilaterally for bilateral carotid occlusion (Chater and Popp 1976, Gratzl et al. 1976, Yonekawa and Yaşargil 1976, Reichmann 1977).

Although such a condition calls for bilateral surgery, the first operation should involve the side that is symptomatically in poorer clinical condition. Prior to the following contralateral operation, the overall situation should be checked once more to determine whether substantial improvement has occurred after the first operation. Holbach

(1977) reports that 11 patients operated upon for unilateral carotid occlusion had improved bilateral EEG results postoperatively. Austin (1974) und Schmiedek (1976) also observed a significant increase in CBF after unilateral anastomosis. Yonekawa and Yaşargil (1976) even mention the case of a patient with a four-vessel occlusion whose postoperative clinical condition was decisively better after extra-intracranial anas-

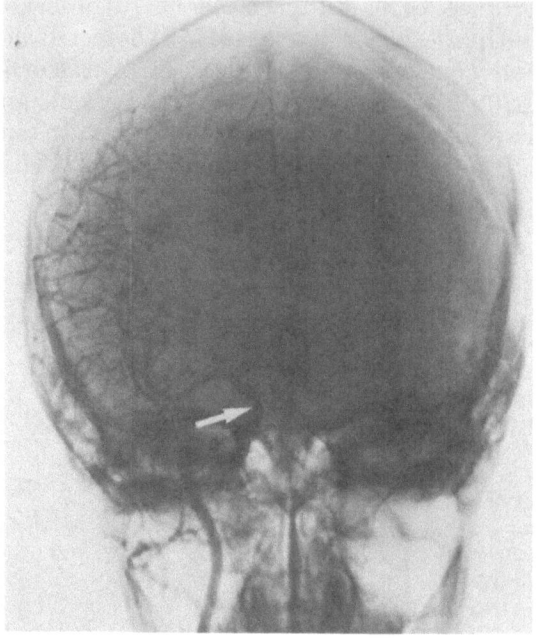

Fig. 81. Right side angiogram of the patient shown in Fig. 74, 1 year after a left side extra-intracranial bypass operation. There is also a stenosis on the right side in the region of the internal carotid artery at a site corresponding to that in the left internal carotid artery

tomosis. This improvement is due to the steal phenomenon; because of it, in certain cases the patient does not require another operation on the contralateral side.

11.6.1. Carotid Occlusion and Contralateral Carotid Stenosis

This combination of multiple vascular lesions is found quite often. Of 80 extra-intracranial anastomoses, it was evidenced in 12 cases (Table 6). A distinction must be made between stenosis in the extracranial and intracranial regions.

If a stenosis is found in the extracranial region, it must be eliminated while a reconstruction is performed by means of extra-intracranial

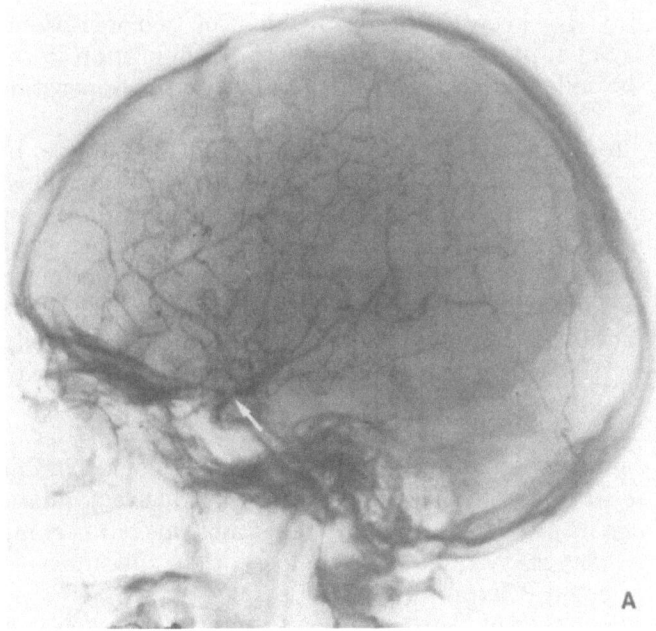

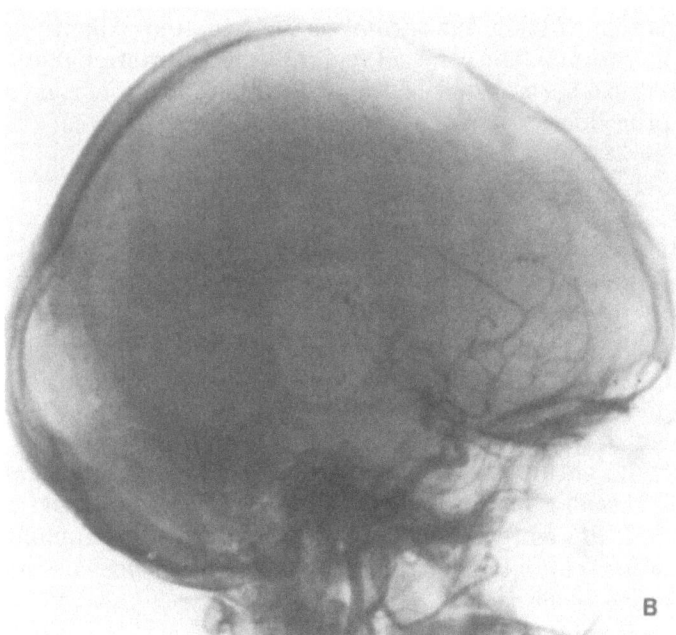

Fig. 82. A) Preoperative high-grade stenosis of the left internal carotid artery in the intracranial part (see also Fig. 75 and Chapter 13). B) High-grade stenosis in the right internal carotid artery

anastomosis in the side of the carotid occlusion. There is no doubt about this procedure. However, the order in which the two operations are to be carried out is not fully clarified: either stenosis operation in the cervical region may be followed by extra-intracranial bypass operation, or vice versa.

Usually, in patients with the condition described above, both brain hemispheres are supplied mostly through the stenosed side. This situation gives rise to certain difficulties during the operation. The clamping time should not exceed 3 minutes. Thus the procedure chosen is usually the following: first, an extra-intracranial anastomosis is performed on the occluded side. This is followed by the operation on the carotid stenosis by a direct extracranial approach. At this stage, additional blood supply of the brain via the extra-intracranial anastomosis is ensured (Spetzler 1978).

At the Department of Neurosurgery, Vienna, this procedure occasionally gave rise to complications (described in detail in Chapter 13). Similar complications are mentioned in the literature available on this subject, which, however, does not take into account complications provoked by extra-intracranial anastomosis or changes in the blood flow of the area affected (Chapter 13).

At the Department of Neurosurgery, the stenosis of the carotid artery in the cervical region is first eliminated surgically. The intraoperative clamping time must be as short as possible. This requires the use of an intraluminar shunt while the thrombus is eliminated. About 8 to 10 days after the operation in the cervical region, extra-intracranial anastomosis is performed. No severe complications were found to occur in connection with this procedure.

11.7. Moya-Moya Syndrome

In 1901 Tandler described the so-called "rete mirabile caroticum" that can be observed in chronic carotid occlusions. It is characterized by the appearance of multiple, although insufficient collaterals which compensate for the vascular deficiencies. In 1961, the same syndrome was observed by Takeuchi in Japanese children. In 1969, it was described as the moya-moya syndrome by Suzuki et al. This syndrome consists of the development of collateral anastomotic pathways in the base of the brain associated with chronic progressive stenosis of the carotid fork. It is not a congenital vascular malformation. This specific radiological syndrome presents clinically as recurring cerebrovascular insults in children or as recurrent subarachnoid hemorrhage in adults; it has been described in all races including black.

Surgery involving cervical sympathectomy and cervical ganglion-ectomy was rarely successful prior to the introduction of extra-intracranial anastomosis. In 1975 Krayenbühl reported for the first time the case of a 4-year-old boy who was subjected to extra-intracranial anastomosis for moya-moya. In spite of the boy's unfavorable initial condition, he made a very good recovery, and the neurological deficits regressed almost completely. Although this syndrome has a rather low incidence, several cases were described in the following years in which satisfactory recovery was achieved by extra-intracranial anastomosis (Mastri 1973, Heilbrunn 1974, Austin 1975, Kikuchi 1975, Reichmann 1975, Numaguchi *et al.*, Tamin 1976, Yonekawa and Yaşargil 1976). In 1977, Amine reported one

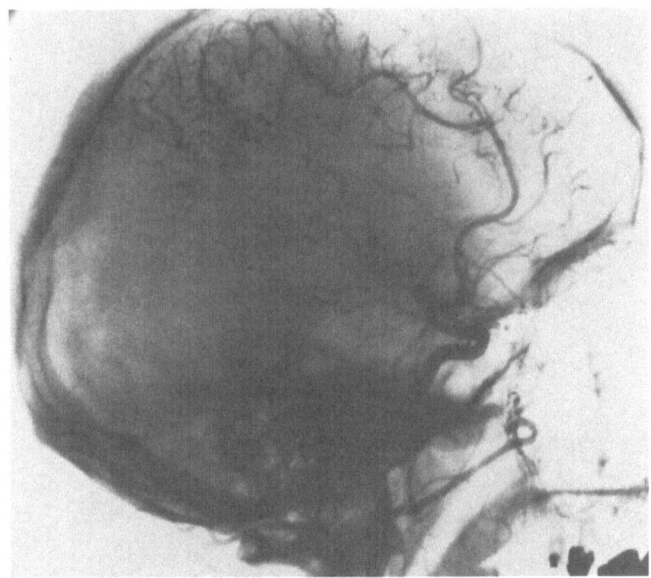

Fig. 83. Moya-moya syndrome in a 47-year-old patient (case 58) with a left sided hemiparesis. The small enlarged collaterals in the parietal region and near the trunk of the middle cerebral artery are clearly visible

case of bilateral extra-intracranial bypass for moya-moya in both hemispheres of the brain.

Reichmann (1975) expressed the opinion that the very satisfactory improvement noticed after such operations was mainly due to a change in blood flow conditions. This was confirmed by Heilbrunn (1974). He performed rCBF measurement in two cases of moya-moya both pre- and postoperatively. The theory of blood flow changes is supported by the fact that the small collaterals characteristic of moya-moya may disappear after extra-intracranial anastomosis. Figure 83 shows the angiogram of a 47-year-old patient with an occlusion of the middle cerebral artery and insufficient perfusion of the middle cerebral artery region by minute collaterals arising from the area supplied by the anterior cerebral artery. There was a considerable regression of these small collaterals 8 days

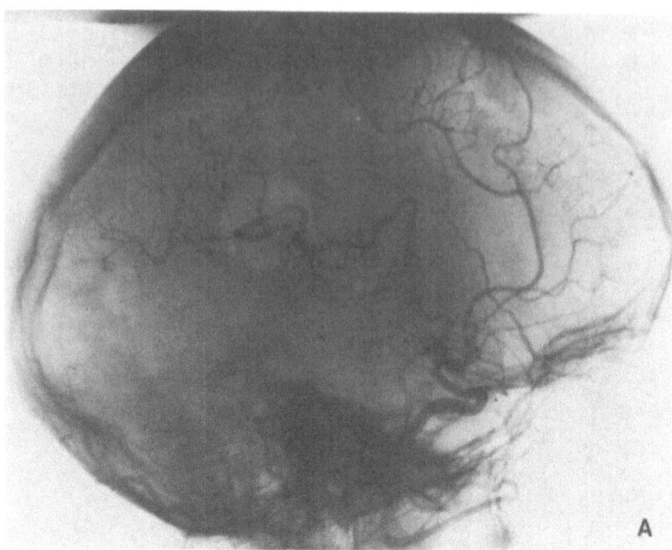

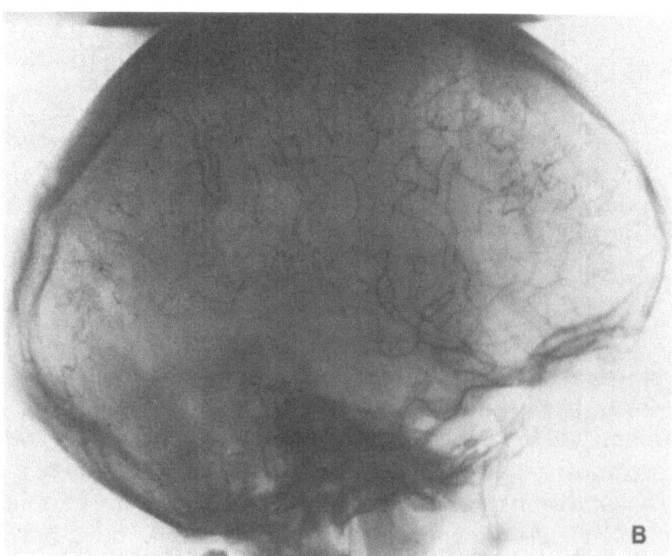

Fig. 84. A) Angiogram of patient shown in Fig. 83 8 days postoperatively. Function of the anastomosis is very satisfactory with a very good supply to the middle cerebral artery region. B) At the later stages the small pathological collaterals are no longer visible

postoperatively (Fig. 84). The patient also recovered from the hemiparesis a few days after the operation.

Before the introduction of extra-intracranial anastomosis at the Department of Neurosurgery, Vienna, a case of moya-moya was observed in a 35-year-old patient. The hemiplegia on the left side had not improved after 3 years.

In the author's opinion, the small collaterals are at least partly able to ensure the blood supply to the area cut off from regular circulation. They are insufficient, however, to ensure undisturbed functioning of the damaged region. Only extra-intracranial anastomosis can restore the blood flow to this region, even if it is performed at a later stage. The collateral circulation, however insignificant it may be, keeps the area functioning to a certain extent. Angiographic results revealing the regression of the small collaterals further substantiate the theory that blood flow changes have taken place. Extra-intracranial anastomosis is the first really satisfactory and successful treatment for this rare syndrome.

11.8. Vascular Malformations

11.8.1. Aneurysms

Large aneurysms continue to be a major problem in neurosurgery because in some few cases it may not be possible to operate upon without causing an occlusion of a large cerebral vessel or of the internal carotid artery. Frequently, permanent severe neurological deficits are the result of such operations. In recent years, some aneurysms were successfully operated upon by means of extra-intracranial anastomosis (Yaşargil 1970, Reichmann 1975, Yonekawa and Yaşargil 1975, Chater 1976, Ammermann and Smith 1977, Deruty 1977). The number of published cases is small because two highly difficult techniques are simultaneously involved in this procedure: aneurysm surgery must be preceded by extra-intracranial anastomosis. The anastomosis must begin functioning immediately after the operation on the aneurysm and the occluded vessel. It would be meaningless to perform extra-intracranial anastomosis a few weeks before the surgical treatment of the aneurysm. The anastomosis would only occlude during that period because of the absence of a pressure gradient under normal blood flow conditions (Yaşargil 1973). The results reported thus far justify the efforts and difficulties associated with this procedure (Figs. 85 and 86).

Figure 85 shows the angiogram of a 46-year-old women with a big aneurysm and occlusion of a branch of the middle cerebral artery. Figure 86 shows the clipped aneurysm and the extra-intracranial anastomosis.

11.8.2. Angiomas

Deruty (1974) performed an extra-intracranial anastomosis preceding the extirpation of an arteriovenous angioma. Because a major vessel

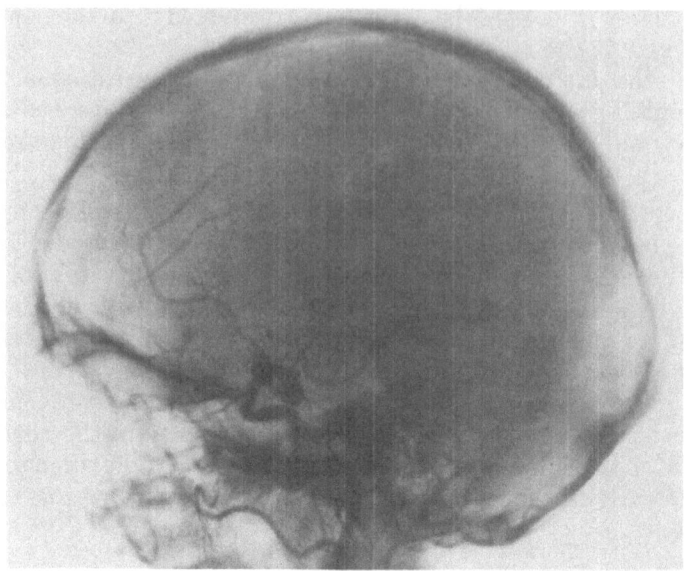

Fig. 85. A 46-year-old female patient (case 5) with a large, sack-shaped aneurysm of the posterior communicating artery, an occlusion of the middle cerebral artery, and right sided high-grade hemiparesis and somnolence

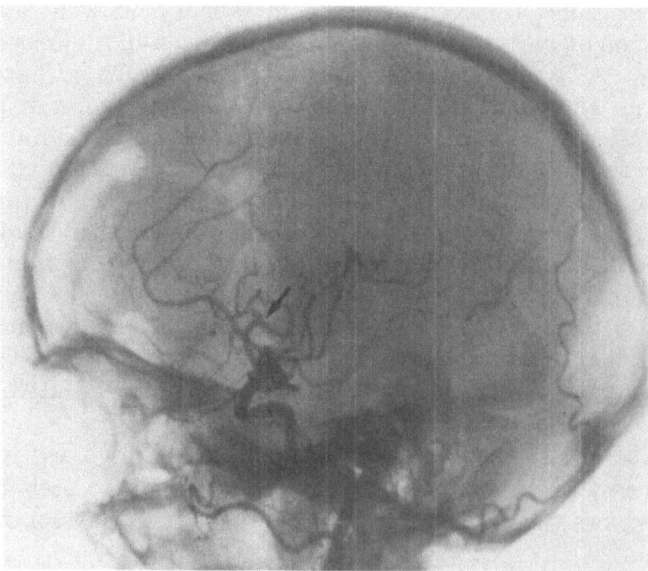

Fig. 86. Postoperative angiogram made 10 days after operation in patient shown in Fig. 85 shows the Yaşargil clip applied to the aneurysm and that the extra-intracranial bypass operation performed at the same time is functioning well (arrow)

can occasionally be clamped during extirpation, an extra-intracranial anastomosis can improve the vascularization in the involved area.

In a 44-year-old patient large arteriovenous angioma was detected angiographically in the left temporoparietal region following sub-arachnoid hemorrhage (Fig. 87). Postoperatively, the patient had hemiplegia on the right side, accompanied by an almost complete aphasia.

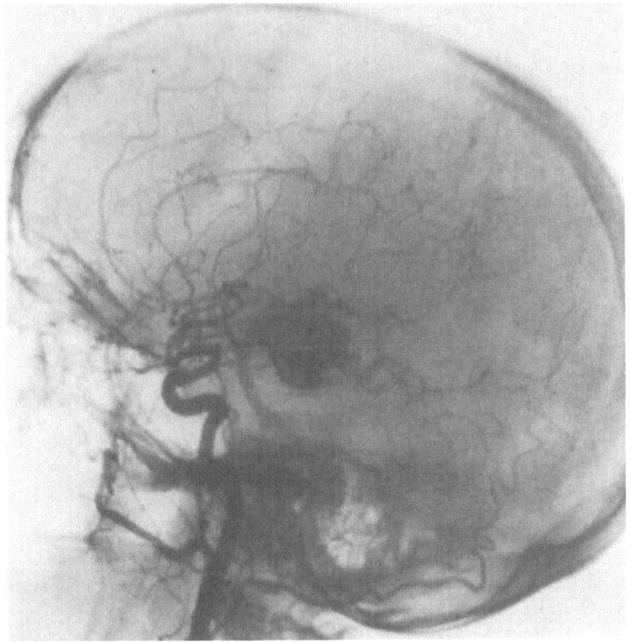

Fig. 87. A 44-year-old female patient with large arteriovenous angioma in the left temporal region (case 14)

Follow-up angiography revealed an occlusion of the middle cerebral artery (Fig. 88 A). Extra-intracranial anastomosis was performed with the occipital artery 16 days after the first operation. Hemiplegia and aphasia receded 1 week postoperatively. Follow-up angiography showed the irrigation of the middle cerebral artery region via the occipital anastomosis (Fig. 88 B).

11.9. Other Indications

Carotid cavernous fistulas are another indication for extra-intracranial anastomosis. An occlusion of the internal carotid artery can be caused by almost any surgical procedure on such fistulas.

Large benign *tumors* are also a surgical indication. The extirpation of such tumors may cause a lesion of a large vessel (Fig. 89) and extra-intracranial bypass operation can prevent neurological deficit.

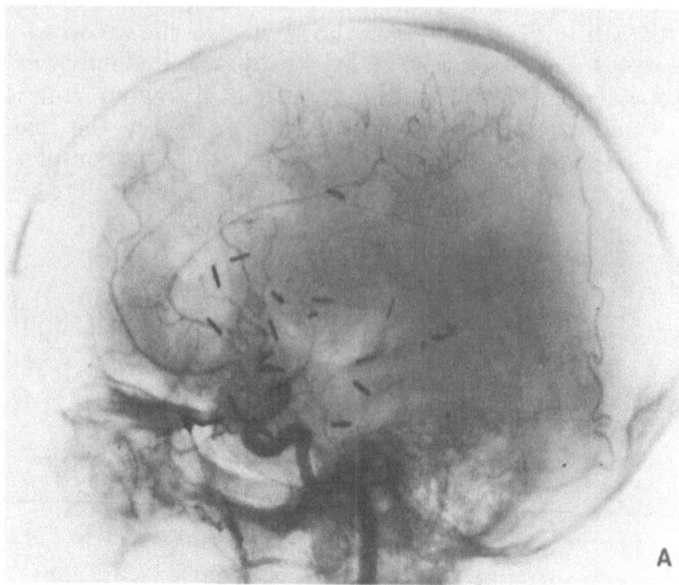

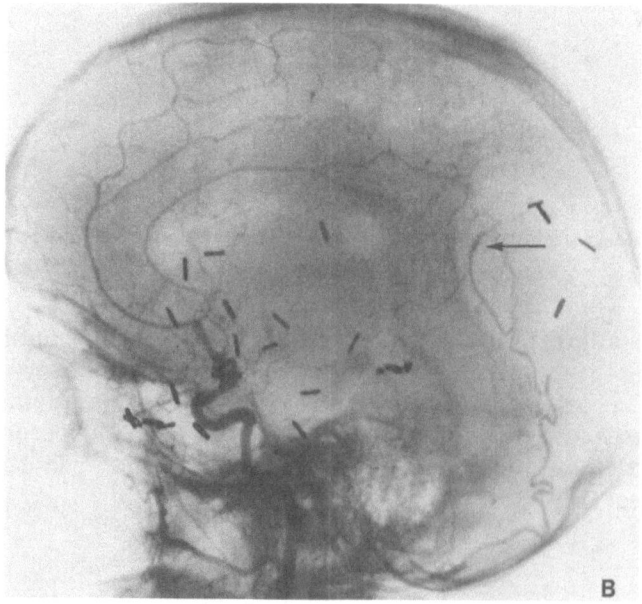

Fig. 88. A) The middle cerebral artery is closed by a clip during extirpation of the angioma. The occipital artery is well represented. B) Extra-intracranial anastomosis is performed 7 days after the angioma operation between the occipital artery and a branch of the middle cerebral artery. The occipital artery is somewhat dilated and the angular region is moderately irrigated

11.10. Traumatic Vascular Lesions

Traumatic vascular lesions—for example occlusion of the carotid artery in the neck or in the base of skull—are very often accompanied by severe neurological deficits. Unlike sclerotic occlusions, they set in suddenly and, there is no time for the collaterals to adapt to the changed conditions. As a rule, indication for surgery will depend on the location of

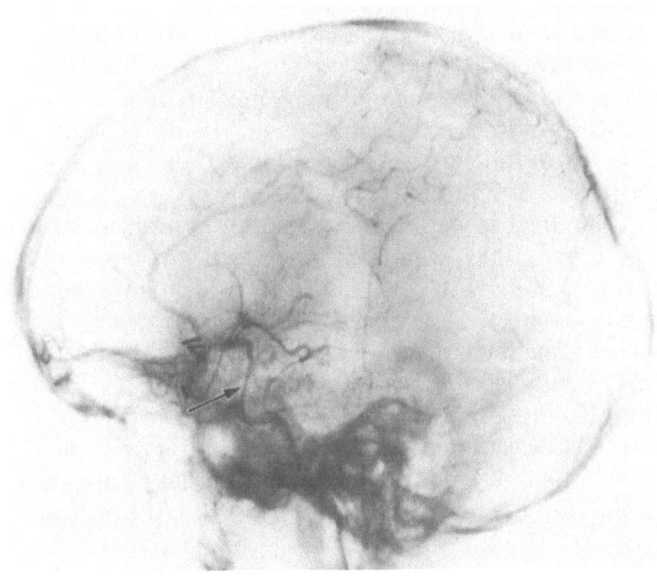

Fig. 89. A 16-year-old patient who had surgery on a meningioma at the basis of the skull and then experienced a relapse. The internal carotid artery is severly stenosed for a length of about 1 cm. This situation is a good indication for extra-intracranial anastomosis

the lesions and the type of neurological deficit. As in the case of acute carotid occlusions in the cervical region, the question is whether to operate at the acute stage, provided that the patient is available for surgery a few hours after the event. Although acute reconstructive surgery on the afferent brain vessels has occasionally been successful (Gratzl *et al.* 1976), the risk of a postoperative cerebral edema is too great to justify surgery for an acute vascular occlusion (Kletter 1978).

Vascular occlusions should be operated upon no sooner than 3 weeks after they appear. Surgery should be preceded by scintigraphy, CBF measurement, and computerized tomography of the cerebral parenchyma in the damaged area. Gratzl *et al.* (1975), who operated on traumatic vascular lesions, arrived at the same conclusions.

12. Indications for Extra-Intracranial Bypass Procedure: Clinical Aspects

12.1. Transient Ischemic Attacks (Transient Cerebral Ischemia)

A transient ischemic attack (TIA) is a focal disturbance of the cerebral circulation, often recurrent, that causes impaired function lasting a short period of time which then recovers without residual disability. The shortest attack is only a few seconds long, most attacks last an average of 10 to 20 minutes, and others last for several hours. The duration of the attack, within the definition, is arbitrary; most authors, however, accept a maximum period of 24 hours.

Transient cerebral ischemia is a common symptom with an annual incidence of 2 per 1000 population between the ages of 65 and 74 (Whisnant 1974). Men with TIA outnumber women except in the age group over 80.

A TIA in the area of the internal carotid artery is the result of occlusive (Fischer 1951, Fields et al. 1968), stenotic (Wolsey and Jandruck 1973), and embolic (Fischer 1959, Fields et al. 1970) vascular phenomena. Comprehensive statistics suggest that up to 50 percent of the patients suffering a completed stroke had TIA in their case history. This emphasizes the importance of detecting these TIA. The most important

Table 7. *Most Important Functional Disorders Associated With TIA*

Region of Internal Carotid Artery	Region of Vertebral Artery
Visual uniocular loss	Vertigo
Amaurosis fugax	Ataxia
Weakness of arm and/or leg	Disturbance of consciousness
Paraesthesiae	Dysarthria
Speech disturbances	Diplopia
Facial paresis	Oscillopsia
Focal convulsive seizures	Movement of the field of vision
Sensory loss	Epileptic seizures
	Headache

functional disorders associated with TIA are listed in Table 7. The preoperative examinations mentioned in Chapter 7 are absolutely required whenever TIA is suspected. If the patient has an operable lesion—i.e., either an extracranial or an intracranial lesion eligible for extra-intracranial anastomosis—then surgery is a must, otherwise he runs a greater risk of having a stroke. Table 11, page 124, lists the patients with a completed stroke upon whom extra-intracranial anastomosis was performed at the Department of Neurosurgery, Vienna, in 1975 and 1976. Many of them had multiple transient ischemic attacks before the stroke.

The data on the sites of arterial narrowing and occlusion found on four vessel angiography in patients with transient ischemia are taken from a cooperative study. The frequency of stenotic lesions in cases of TIA at the origin of the internal carotid (33.8 percent) and the vertebral artery (20 percent) is high; 19.4 percent of patients showed no occlusion and 6.1 percent showed intracranial vascular lesions (Haas et al. 1968). In patients with carotid occlusion, propagation of the thrombus proceeds throughout the artery so that it is impossible to determine the original site of occlusion. The high proportion of multiple lesions (67.3 percent) is important and has a bearing both on pathogenesis and treatment. Detailed clarification is also necessary in order to differentiate TIA from focal epilepsy, migraine, hypoglycemia associated with diabetes (Meier and Portnoi 1958), and peripheral labyrinthopathy.

12.1.1. Preoperative Examinations

Electroencephalography is absolutely required after a TIA in addition to routine examinations, such as measurement of peripheral blood pressure and blood tests. Although following a TIA the EEG is asymptomatic, it is nonetheless of importance in determining epileptic seizures.

After a TIA *cerebral scintigraphy* also does not provide pathological findings; but, like the EEG, it is also required in order to exclude various gradual processes.

Doppler sonography is also a very important test method. One must remember that the vessel portion beyond the bifurcation of the ophthalmic artery from the internal carotid artery cannot be evaluated, however there is only a 10 percent probability of a lesion being located distally from the ophthalmic artery.

Four-vessel angiography is the most important examination method in recognizing the cause of TIA. If angiography does not reveal pathological findings, surgery is definitely contraindicated. The patient, however, should be re-examined regularly. In particular, the chance that an embolization of sclerotic changes in greater depth may have occurred should be kept in mind. An angiography of the aortic arch is then required in order to check the bifurcations of the large vessels leading from the aortic arch, especially if the TIA recur. In such a case, changes in the cardiac valves may also have taken place.

rCBF measurement is of essential importance for the verification of TIA (Gratzl et al. 1976, Austin et al. 1977, Schmiedek et al. 1977).

Although repeated TIAs and clear morphological findings are an indication for a bypass operation, rCBF measurements can clarify two decisive factors: 1. The exact location of the low perfusion area and 2. The degree of low perfusion. Thus the anastomosis can be performed precisely in the damaged area. In doubtful cases, rCBF measurements may be used to verify whether or not low perfusion exists. This is particularly important whenever a TIA occurred recently without recurrent attacks but with angiographically evident vascular changes (Chapter 7, Fig. 41).

Although rCBF measurement is not absolutely required for diagnosing TIA and for establishing the indication for this operation, it is an examination that provides further reliable data and can indicate postoperatively to what extent CBF has improved. In all of 10 reported cases of TIA and rCBF measurement, Gratzl (1976) reduced these attacks with extra-intracranial anastomosis. In 8 patients, rCBF measurements were performed pre- and postoperatively; in all the cases, blood flow was reduced before the operation. In 5 patients CBF reached a substantially higher level immediately postoperatively, with the bypass functioning in all cases.

rCBF measurement is the only method that enables diagnoses of a focal reduction of the blood flow and accurate measurement of the postoperative increase in blood flow. The drawback of this method is that only the external carotid artery or, whenever possible, the superficial temporal artery must be perfused with xenon at its trunk by catheter angiography or puncture. This test method not only strains the patient but also is occasionally hazardous (Schmiedek et al. 1976).

At the Department of Neurosurgery, Vienna, rCBF measurement is performed only before operations. Postoperatively, a direct puncture of the temporal artery or visualization with a catheter is considered difficult and dangerous for the patient (Schmiedek et al. 1976). Only in special cases—for example, recurring TIA—should the cause and degree of blood flow be accurately determined. In such cases, we consider rCBF measurement to be absolutely indicated postoperatively. It must be further emphasized, however, that the rCBF method can hardly be employed on a routine basis in the preoperative evaluation of all the potential candidates for bypass surgery.

In patients with TIA, preoperative computerized tomography has been of relatively little use (Schmiedek et al. 1978, Spetzler et al. 1978). Scans have either been normal or have shown only minimal abnormalities. In 22 patients examined by Schmiedek (1978) with angiography, rCBF measurement, and computerized tomography, 15 scans were normal. Low perfusion may be diagnosed only at the time of the attack and a few hours afterward. Thus computerized tomography is not essential for the diagnosis and the indication of extra-intracranial bypass in TIA. It could only be used in addition to EEG and cerebral scintigraphy to exclude other pathological processes.

Postoperative computerized tomography scans have been unchanged in cases of bypass operation.

12.1.2. Conclusion (Preoperative Examinations in TIA)

In order to make a diagnosis of TIA and to establish an indication for surgery, the case history as well as the neurological and the morphological findings, which are obtained by four-vessel angiography, are of major importance. Furthermore, rCBF measurements should be performed in order to obtain objective data concerning the reduction of the blood flow in a given area.

The procedure to be used in diagnosis and treatment is shown in Table 8. Other methods, such as scintigraphy, computerized tomography, and EEG, can be applied primarily to exclude other processes.

Table 8. *Diagnostic Procedures in TIA*

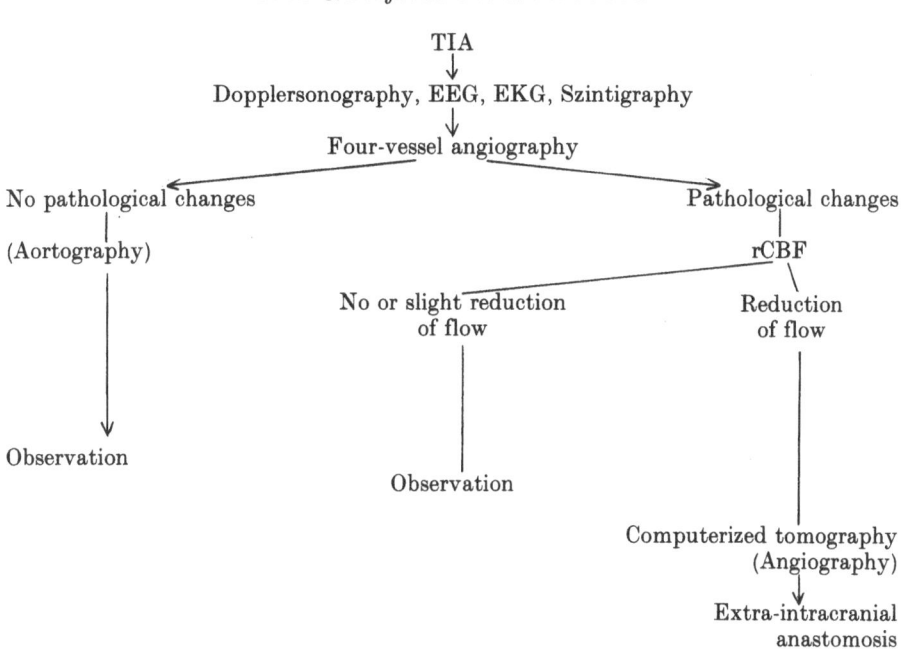

12.1.3. Timing of Operation

In TIA further attacks or completed stroke may follow shortly. Thus, once this vascular lesion has been unequivocally evidenced by angiography, surgery must definitely be planned. The timing, however, must be based on the patient's case history. If there is no doubt that he had only one TIA, the patient should have a general internal examination, since the morphological lesion may not account for the TIA. On the other hand, if the case history includes several attacks, perhaps succeeding each other at short intervals, the operation should be performed within the shortest possible time.

12.1.4. Results of Operation and Postoperative Examinations

The operation is considered successful if no further TIA occur. The improved CBF that is then achieved can be demonstrated by the following methods: observation of the clinical symptoms, angiography, direct observation of the anastomosis and the region supplied by the anastomosis, and rCBF measurement. The last method usually reveals a postoperative increase in rCBF provided that the indication and surgical technique were correct (Chater 1976, Gratzl *et al.* 1976, Ito *et al.* 1977, Schmiedek *et al.* 1977, Deruty *et al.* 1978).

The rate of improvement after an extra-intracranial bypass operation for TIA is between 80 percent (Yonekawa and Yaşargil 1976) and 100 percent (Gratzl 1976). Table 9 provides a survey of the major publications dealing with TIA and the results achieved by extra-intracranial bypass. In our own study of the 27 patients suffering from TIA, 23 were asymptomatic after anastomosis.

Table 9. *Results of Extra-Intracranial Anastomosis in TIA and PRIND*

Author	No.	Im-proved (No TIA)	Un-changed	Worse (late Stroke)	Dead	Patency of Anastomoses
Gratzl *et al.* 1976	29 (65)	29				
Yonekawa and Yaşargil 1976	22 (63)	18				
Samson *et al.* 1977	31 (31)	23	5	3		28 (31)
Chater *et al.* 1978	95 (140)	79				
Kikuchi and Karasawa 1978	16 (113)	15				
Merei and Bodosi 1978	4 (90)	4				
Author's study	27 (100)	23	2	1	1	17 (18)

In reference to TIA, it must be emphasized that cerebrovascular disease associated with arteriosclerosis is a generalized affliction with progressive development. Improvement of the afflicted brain hemisphere is therefore of primary concern. Since TIA develops progressively, further attacks may occur later in the contralateral hemisphere.

Overall morbidity can also be influenced to a decisive extent since an extra-intracranial bypass can also have repercussions on the contralateral hemisphere (Chater 1976). The postoperative morbidity rate in Chater's study is 26 percent. In the author's study, it slightly exceeded 20 percent. This means that the morbidity rate is reduced by two-thirds, of one takes into account that there is a 60 percent probability that TIA patients will have a manifest stroke within 1 year. More exact data will only be obtained when a larger statistical sample exists after a period of approximately 20 years (see Table 13).

12.1.5. Conclusion (TIA and Bypass Operation)

Extra-intracranial anastomosis is a perfect method for the treatment of TIA in the presence of an evident morphological change. On the average, there is no recurrence of TIA in about 90 percent of all patients (Table 10).

12.2. Prolonged Reversible Ischemic Neurological Deficit (PRIND or RIND)

Between a TIA and a stroke, there is a type of attack that appears at first to be a stroke but the neurological deficit subsides completely within 2 to 7 days. This attack is too long in duration to be categorized as a TIA and is different from a completed stroke because it is reversible within short time. RIND is considered as intermediate between TIA and stroke and is to be treated as a forerunner of stroke. This type of stroke corresponds to TIA as far as preoperative diagnostics and treatment are concerned. The preoperative diagnostic methods used are approximately the same as in TIA. Unlike TIA however, EEG, computerized tomography, and scintigraphy can give modifications for low perfusion in the damaged area in RIND. The indication for surgery and the postoperative examinations are the same as in TIA (Chapter 12.1.).

12.3. Completed Stroke

Despite the frequency of stroke, the term itself is a source of confusion. For many people the term "stroke" is synonymous with "hemiplegia", and in the absence of the latter a diagnosis of stroke is not made. This usage ignores the fact that vascular lesions may affect any part of the central nervous system so that an isolated hemianopia, dysphasia, or a focal brain stem lesion may also have a vascular cause. Equally, equating stroke and hemiplegia does not take into account the fact that there are many causes of a hemiplegia other than a circulatory disturbance. A stroke is therefore best defined as a focal neurological persistent deficit due to a vascular lesion which reaches its peak in less than 6 hours.

The final fate of the damaged zone, as well as the patient's condition, depends on the number of collaterals formed, their adaptability, and other factors, such as age, blood pressure, and degree of existing degenerative changes (for example, in arteriosclerosis).

In an occlusion of a great vessel the few existing collaterals apparently

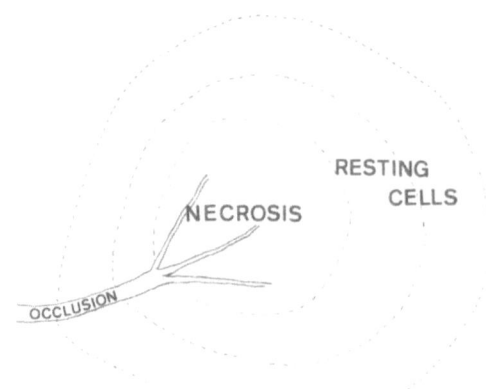

A

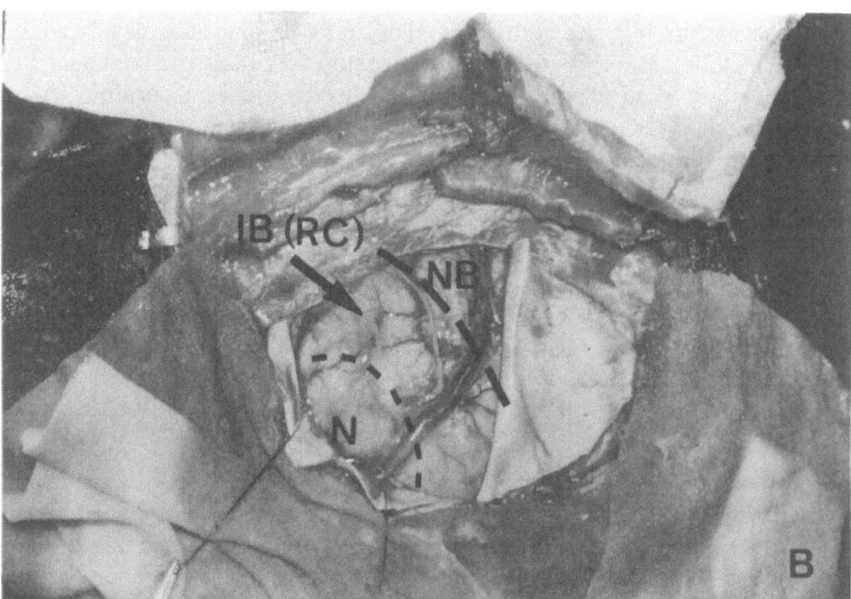

B

Fig. 90. The center of a recently infarcted area usually consists of a necrotic zone (*N*). This is surrounded by a marginal zone of ganglion cells which survive but cannot fulfill their specific function (ischemic brain—*IB*). During the first weeks there is a large edema zone around these "resting ganglion cells" (*RC*). That is about seven times as large the area of the resting ganglion cells. *NB* normal brain

do not prevent neurological deficits. The blood supply to the ischemic region via the collaterals is sufficient, however, to ensure the survival of the damaged cells, at least temporarily. The center of a recently infarcted area usually consists of a necrotic zone. This is surrounded by a marginal zone of ganglion cells that survive but cannot fulfill their specific function. During the first weeks there is a large edema zone around these "resting ganglion cells" (Fig. 90). Reconstructive vascular surgery mainly affects these resting cells but can also influence the edema zone. In purely mathematical terms, the necrotic center portion has the smallest mass, whereas the main mass consists of the intact cells and the edema zone. For example, if the infarcted area is 1 cm in diameter and the area with the resting cells extends, 1 cm around it, the size of the resting cell area is about seven times as large as that of the infarcted area [$V = \frac{4}{3}\pi r^3$: $V = 4\,cm^3$ (infarcted area), $V = 28\,cm^3$ (resting cells)]. In this case, vascular surgery can produce a substantial improvement.

After approximately 3 to 4 weeks, conditions have finally stabilized, so that revascularization can be planned. There is disagreement, however, on whether extra-intracranial anastomosis is indicated in such cases or not. Very often, such operations have not been successful. On the other hand, surprisingly good results have been achieved in other cases. This can be explained by the fact that even with the most sophisticated examination methods it cannot be ascertained with complete accuracy whether or not intact cerebral areas remain that would make an operation worthwhile. At the Department of Neurosurgery, Vienna, we abstain from surgery only if the available findings prove without a doubt the complete destruction of the brain region in question. If there is only a slight chance of improving the patient's condition, we must not forget that a *repeated stroke* may occur; this would then affect the remaining intact area around the completed infarction.

Thus, in a completed stroke, preoperative examinations must try to exclude irreversible cases from surgery.

Unless all examination methods described above are applied, one must remember that the number of patients in whom extra-intracranial anastomosis following a completed stroke will not produce any improvement will be relatively high.

12.3.1. Preoperative Examinations

The investigation of patients suffering from completed stroke seeks to answer a series of questions:

1. Is the patient's neurological problem in fact due to vascular disease, or is some totally different pathology responsible—*e.g.*, tumor, hematoma, epilepsy, multiple sclerosis, *etc.*?

2. What is the anatomy of the vascular lesion? Is the occlusion intracranial or extracranial? Is the source of embolism cardiac or in neck vessels?

3. What stage has the dynamic process reached?

4. Can vascular surgery be considered?

All these questions are important in the management of individual patients, and the examinations supplement the information to be gained about site, pathology, and time course from the history and physical examination (Ross *et al.* 1973).

Acute cerebrovascular lesions are usually accompanied by an abnormality of the surface-recorded *EEG*. A variety of changes may be seen. In a series recorded within 2 weeks of the onset of these lesions, Cohn (1949) found 25 percent of the patients to have a normal record or to show only mild changes. Normal records are common with brain stem vascular lesions.

It is not usually possible to distinguish between cerebral hemorrhage and cerebral infarction. The site of the vascular lesion within the brain may be indicated. As already noted, a focus of delta activity suggests a cortical lesion. On contrast, discordance between the EEG signs and the severity of the hemiplegia is common with an internal capsular lesion. EEG is not of great value in determining indications for surgery.

A completed stroke seldom produces pathologically increased concentrations in cerebral *scintigraphy* during the first 3 to 5 days. Five days after the attack the findings are positive in about 70 to 80 percent of all cases. After the third week the concentration decreases and it is usually no longer detectable 6 to 8 weeks after the attack. This suggests that the concentration of the indicator is linked to repair processes of the cerebral tissue.

The areas showing high scintigraphic concentration largely correspond to the infarcted area. The typical scintigraphic findings of a cerebral stroke are wedgeshaped and correspond to the malacia. The diagnosis cannot clearly differentiate between a cerebral infarction and an intracranial hemorrhage. Therefore, if the findings of cerebral scintigraphy are positive, the examination must be supplemented by angiography. If an apoplectic cerebral tumor is present, the scintigraphic findings will be positive as soon as a few hours after the stroke. In this case cerebral scintigraphy provides for the establishment of a differential diagnosis. It is not possible to draw final conclusions as to the prognosis of the patient.

As described in Chapter 7, *four-vessel angiography* is indispensable if extra-intracranial anastomosis is to be performed. Besides enabling an accurate determination of the morphological changes and the collateral circulations, it also makes it possible to determine the approximate size of the infarcted area. Most important of all, any processes that might be due to intracranial hemorrhage, a tumor, or an edema can be excluded immediately. Thus angiography must be considered the most decisive method of examination from a clinical point of view.

rCBF measurement has a significant role in the examination and definition of the cerebral status in completed stroke.

Both the localization and the degree of the reduced blood flow can be determined by means of rCBF measurements. However, no reliable data can be obtained in cerebral areas that lack all functions. rCBF measurements should be performed in all cases of completed stroke. They are particularly valuable in conjunction with computerized tomography (Schmiedek *et al.* 1978, Spetzler *et al.* 1978). Furthermore, it is possible to establish a preoperative prognosis with regard to the positive or negative functioning of the anastomosis (Schmiedek *et al.* 1976, Austin 1977). If CBF conditions are not good in an area where the anastomosis is to be performed—as in, for example, malacic tissue—then the pressure gradient between the extracranial and intracranial circulations is insufficient and low. This may lead to an occlusion of the anastomosis. If postoperative rCBF measurements are to be performed, then preoperative rCBF measurements become even more meaningful, because then the effect and the functioning of the anastomosis can be even more precisely assessed (Gratzl *et al.* 1976).

The focal reduction of CBF has proved to be an ideal indication for extra-intracranial anastomosis in a completed stroke, because in this case the temporal superficial artery is able to irrigate a defined area. A generalized reduction in CBF—for example, of an entire hemisphere—does not provide a ideal starting point. Nevertheless, even then is it possible to achieve good results by extra-intra-cranial anastomosis (Chater *et al.* 1976, Gratzl *et al.* 1976). A normal CBF may indicate normal conditions—in which case extra-intracranial anastomosis is naturally contraindicated. On the other hand, the results may be negative due to malacic or cystic cerebral tissue. If possible, computerized tomography therefore should be performed in a completed stroke before rCBF measurements are made.

In *computerized tomography* there is usually a correlation between the neurological status and the morphological picture. In a brain that has experienced a completed stroke, however, the findings are positive after a period of 3 to 4 weeks (Chapter 7, Figs. 43, 44). Computerized tomography is absolutely advisable in cases of completed stroke, in particular when numerous neurological symptoms are present. This method allows the immediate elimination of all cases in which surgery is contraindicated or not feasible before any further extensive examination is performed, such as Xenon clearance. The morphological picture of a computer tomogram showing favorable or unfavorable situations for extra-intracranial anastomosis was already described in Chapter 7, Figures 43 to 45. If the findings reveal the presence of a cyst, extra-intracranial anastomosis as well as any further examination in this case is contraindicated. If the density is reduced, even to a large extent, the operation may be performed, but not without taking these findings or rCBF measurements into consideration. If the reduction of density is slight, the operation can definitely be performed.

12.3.2. Conclusion of the Preoperative Examinations (Completed Stroke)

The examination procedure in completed strokes is summarized in Table 10. We believe that in establishing a useful indication, it is important first to eliminate those patients who are not suited for surgery. Among these are (apart from patients with clear contraindications) those who suffer from extensive malacia in combination with a cyst. This diagnosis can rarely be made by angiography alone. Computerized tomography gives a relatively accurate morphological picture and is therefore especially important as a primary tool for selection. If angiography and computerized tomography do not clarify the situation sufficiently, then the decisive method of examination is rCBF measurement (Gratzl et al. 1976, Schmiedek et al. 1976, Austin et al. 1978). The clinical findings are also important as a means of selection, especially since it is not always possible to perform computerized tomography and rCBF measurements.

There is usually a correlation between the tomographic and, clinical findings and the performance of the extra-intracranial anastomosis. In hemiplegic patients the tomography normally shows a big malacic cyst. Extra-intracranial anastomosis cannot improve the neurological deficits of these patients. Good or even excellent results can be achieved in terms of improved neurological symptoms in some patients with only moderate neurological deficits whose tomographic findings show a greater reduction of density in the involved area. If only minor neurological deficits exist, then the tomographic picture shows only a medium reduction of density. Extra-intracranial anastomosis produces excellent results in these cases.

Table 10. *Diagnostic Procedure in Completed Stroke*

Completed Stroke

Four-vessel angiography

EEG   Brain scan

Computerized tomography

Necrosis, Cysts

NO Extra-intracranial   (rCBF measurement)
anastomosis

Extra-intracranial anastomosis

Various examinations were correlated with rCBF measurements and the results were published by Schmiedek in 1978. The rCBF measurements did not show any changes in cases of extensive malacic cysts. The degree in the reduction of density and the degree of the neurological deficits correlated with the degree of reduction in rCBF measurements.

If good results are expected to be achieved with meaningful surgery, the methods of examination should be computerized tomography, four-vessel angiography, and rCBF measurements.

12.3.3. Results of Operation and Postoperative Examinations of Cases With Completed Stroke

As is shown in Table 12, all authors have achieved excellent results with extra-intracranial anastomosis in cases of completed stroke. The question may be raised, however, if the positive results are due to the well-known natural repair and regeneration capacity rather than to the operation itself.

Spontaneous recovery of neurological function after a completed stroke usually occurs within the first 8 weeks. There is no doubt, however, that an immediate relationship exists when the neurological symptoms show an improvement within several days or even hours after the operation. It is more difficult to draw a reliable conclusion if improvement is observed only months after the operation. It should be remembered that extra-intracranial anastomosis establishes a collateral circulation in an affected area. This area can rarely perform the residual functions without the additional blood supply, and if it weren't for the increased supply of oxygen, which is primarily directed toward the area around the existing necrosis (page 118), this area would suffer a complete breakdown in the months following the stroke.

All of the cases reported by Gratzl et al. 1976 were operated on at a much later time. From these results it is concluded that in carefully selected patients with completed strokes it is reasonable to perform an extra-intracranial anastomosis. Patients with severe neurological deficits or a general severe reduction of CBF, however, are poor candidates for surgery; in this group only about 20 percent improved.

Patients with slight or moderate neurological deficits showed good improvement (Tables 11, 12).

In contrast to TIA, in which the operation is considered a success if the attack does not recur and the angiographic evidence does not indicate anastomosic occlusion, the requirement in a completed stroke is an objective improvement in the neurological symptoms. This calls for a more meticulous *postoperative evaluation* process, which comprises several examination methods.

As described in Chapter 7, the *neurological* status has to be determined carefully immediately before and after the operation. This method of examination is the only one that can be performed at all times, even immediately after surgery, without undue discomfort to the patient. With this examination it is possible to objectify any and all improvement in the neurological symptoms. Experience has shown that improvement in neurological deficits postoperatively may indicate further rapid improvement.

The postoperative *neuropsychological examination* is especially

Table 11. *Patients With Completed Stroke (Arrow Downwards), Operated at the Neurosurgical Clinic, Vienna, Over a Period of 2 Years*
Improvement of neurological signs and symptoms (arrow upwards) depends on when the operation was carried out. In some cases of long-time neurological deficiencies there was no postoperative improvement (cases 4, 22, 25). Asterisks indicate the number of TIAs before the stroke

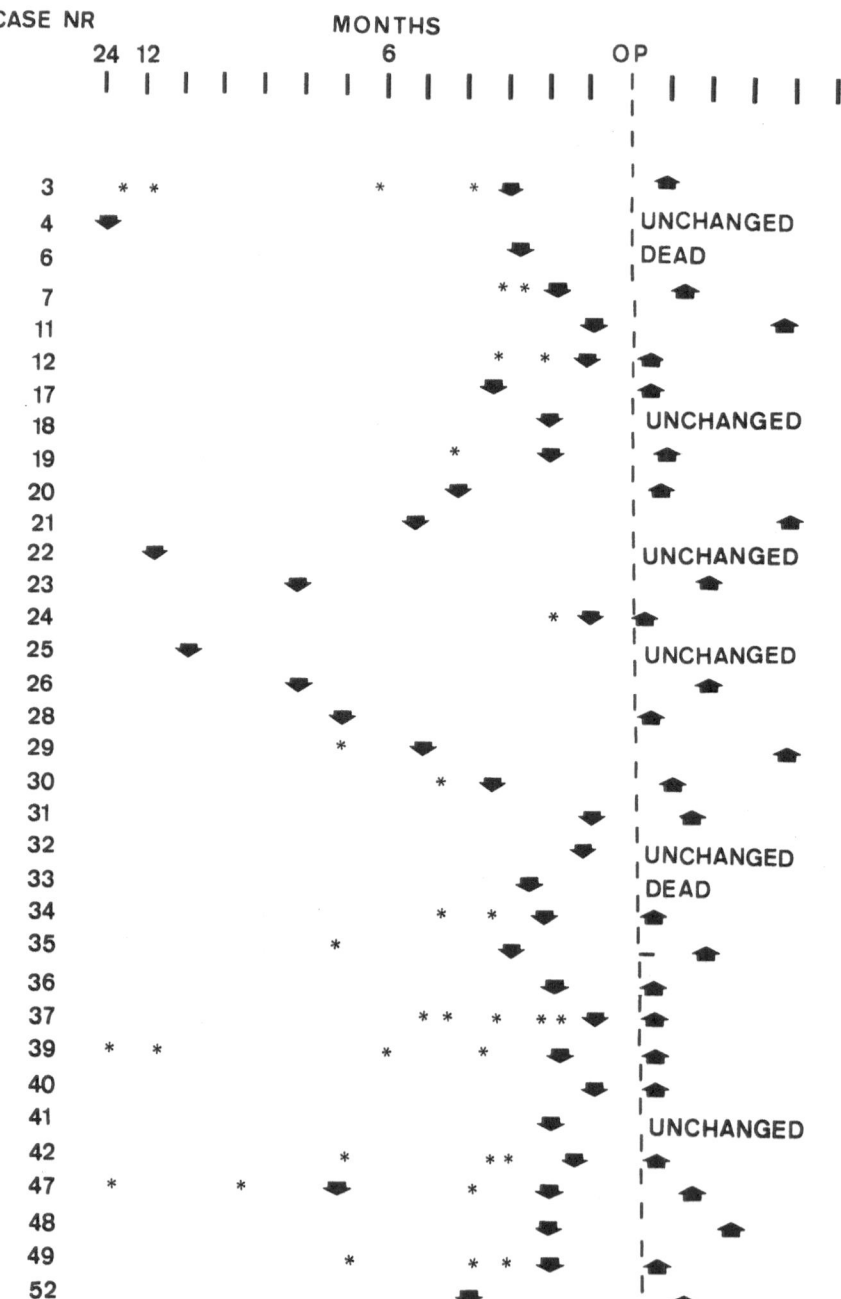

Table 12. *Results of Extra-Intracranial Anastomosis in Cases of Completed Stroke*

Author	No.	Im-proved	Un-changed	Worse	Dead
Chater and Popp 1976	31 (100)				
mild and moderate deficit	25	12			
severe deficit	6	1			
Gratzl *et al.* 1976	29 (65)				
mild and moderate deficit	8	8			
severe deficit	21		20		1
Yonekawa and Yaşargil 1976	39 (63)				
mild and moderate deficit	28	21			
severe deficit	11	5			
Holbach *et al.* 1977	11				
mild and moderate deficit	11	10			1
severe deficit	0				
Kikuchi and Karasawa 1978	86				
mild and moderate deficit	60	30	29		1
severe deficit	26	3	23		5
Merei and Bodosi 1978	86 (90)				
mild and moderate deficit	72	38	30	1	
severe deficit	14	4	10		
Mizukami *et al.* 1978	36				
mild and moderate deficit	17	12	5		
severe deficit	19	1	18		
Author's study	68 (100)				
mild and moderate deficit	51	37 (73%)	9 (17%)	1	4
severe deficit	17	7 (41%)	9 (52%)		1

Table 13. *Patients With Vascular Lesions not Operated (1973)*
(Results one year after stroke)

	No.	Improved	Unchanged	Worse	Dead
TIA	28	7 (25%)	8	4 (39%)	2
C.S.	39				
Mild and moderate deficit	29	9 (31%)	6	12 (41%)	2
Severe deficit	10	2 (20%)	5		3

important in cases of dementia. Its importance in patients with a completed stroke who have undergone extra-intracranial anastomosis has been pointed out by several authors (Austin 1975, Yonekawa and Yaşargil 1975, Evans and Austin 1977, Holbach 1977).

Improvement of the postoperative *EEG* results is usually accompanied by an improvement in the clinical findings, but this is not an essential postoperative examination in cases of completed stroke.

Doppler sonography has no significance as a clinical examination. It can, however, be very useful in evaluating the morphological functioning of the anastomosis (Hofmann *et al.* 1978).

Since cerebral *scintigraphy* primarily indicates transformation processes (Chapter 7.5.), it has no importance in postoperative examinations in cases of completed strokes.

Cerebral *angiography* is indispensable because it aids in evaluating the functioning of the anastomosis, just as it does in cases of TIA. If areas still exist that have not been irreversibly damaged in the affected brain area, and if the anastomosis was performed satisfactorily, the superficial temporal artery will show a dilatation within a few days. If severe brain damage exists, which is often recognizable intraoperatively, then postoperative angiography will show no dilatation in the superficial temporal artery. Another important fact is that with angiography it is possible to diagnose any change in the collateral circulation system (Chapter 13).

Computerized tomography is also of decisive importance as a postoperative examination because it is a noninvasive procedure. With this examination—provided that the anastomosis is functioning satisfactorily and the demand for blood is supplied—it is possible to register an increase in density in a low-density area as early as a few weeks after the operation (Spetzler *et al.* 1978).

In regard to postoperative flow, *rCBF measurement* is also an essential method of examination. It cannot be routinely performed, however, because accurate evaluation requires direct puncture of the superficial temporal artery, which may then jeopardize the entire operation (Schmiedek *et al.* 1978). An extensive series of studies made by Austin (1976) and Schmiedek *et al.* (1976, 1978) indicate, however, that improved neurological symptoms, satisfactory angiographic results, and improved computerized tomography findings correlate with a clear increase in regional and to some extent an increase in global CBF in all cases.

Conclusion

The most important postoperative examinations performed in cases of a completed stroke are regular short-term check-ups of the neurological status and neuropsychological examinations. Four-vessel angiography is of prime importance in cases of a completed stroke. Computerized tomography should also be performed if possible. Satisfactory objective results can be obtained by rCBF measurements with xenon, although this method is not suitable as a routine examination. All the other postoperative examination methods are only of secondary importance.

12.3.4. Conclusion (Completed Stroke and Bypass Operation)

Although in individual cases extra-intracranial anastomosis in completed stroke has been justly denied credit for the improvement of the neurological symptoms, there is no doubt that patients suffering from a slight or medium-grade neurological deficit may improve considerably. Accurate preoperative diagnostice evaluation—aimed mainly at sparing those patients an operation who may not expect a neurological improvement due to the lack of brain parenchyma—is prerequisite for surgery in cases of completed stroke. A large percentage of those patients who have not suffered a severe deficit following a completed stroke may resume work. Extra-intracranial anastomosis is an ideal surgical treatment for completed stroke and slight or medium-grade neurological deficit due to morphological changes that have been inoperable up to now (see Table 11, page 124, Tables 12, 13, page 125).

12.4. Progressive Stroke (Stroke in Evolution)

A progressive stroke is defined as a persistent deficit that takes 6 hours to several days to reach its maximum. The onset of neurological deficits can occur progressively or stepwise. The clinical picture corresponds more or less to that of a manifest stroke, and in principle it is greatly related to the latter. There is, however, one difference, which is related to the timing of the operation.

If a patient has rapidly progressing neurological symptoms, and if the presence of a visible pathological change is confirmed (for example, occlusion of a middle cerebral artery or the internal carotid artery), the surgeon must decide whether an immediate operation can influence the patient's deteriorating condition. In such a case extra-intracranial anastomosis is performed at the acute phase and is only occasionally successful. Gratzl (1976) reports that of 7 patients who had surgery for a stroke in evolution, 5 patients expired postoperatively and the condition of the remaining 2 patients deteriorated. Yonekawa (1976) reports 2 cases in which the patients' condition improved slightly after the operation. At the Department of Neurosurgery, Vienna, 4 patients were operated on for a stroke in evolution; two of them died a short time after operation. In two cases the condition improved immediatly after operation.

Weinstein (1978) reports six patients who were operated on a progressive stroke. In four patients who underwent surgical treatment within 10 and 3 days after the appearance of neurological symptoms a slight improvement could be noticed, but these patients were unable to go back to work. Two patients whose neurological deficits had lasted for as long as 3 months improved enough to be able to work again.

This discrepancy between the various experiences of the authors performing operations in cases of progressive stroke can be explained by the fact that all *patients died who showed progressive neurological symptoms within a few hours and were operated on only a few hours later*. In general, better results were achieved in those cases in which the neurological symptoms appeared less rapidly and the operation was performed a few days later. Good results were achieved in retarded progressive strokes, which may, however, be treated as completed strokes, as the distinction between the two is blurred.

Although the causes of the postoperative deterioration noted in some cases are not completely clear, the occurrence of the first clinical symptoms following a vascular occlusion indicates a severe disorder in the affected cerebral matter and the surrounding area. There is an imbalance in particular of the blood-cerebrospinal fluid barrier, and any increase in blood flow at this stage (as caused by an operation for acute stroke) is followed by severe cerebral edema. This has been confirmed by postmortem examinations (Gratzl 1974, Meyermann *et al.* 1978).

On the basis of the clinical results following vascular surgery for progressive stroke, a distinction must be made between *1. rapid progressive stroke* (duration of 6 to 24 hours to reach the maximum of persistent deficit) and *2. retarded progressive stroke* (duration of more than 24 hours to reach the maximum of persistent deficit). The limit between these two categories cannot be exactly defined due to the small number of cases published thus far, although it is assumed to be approximately 24 hours.

According to the literature and this author's experience, surgery of a *rapid progressive stroke* (severe neurological deficits appearing within a few hours) *is in any event contraindicated. In a retarded progressive stroke*, on the other hand, *extra-intracranial anastomosis is indicated.*

12.5. Generalized Low-Perfusion Syndrome

This syndrome has seldom been described (Yonekawa and Yaşargil 1975, Chater 1976). It is characterized by a general deterioration of the functional capacity of the brain, marked by a certain lack of stimulation and frontal symptoms. Focal deficits need not necessarily be present. These individuals may complain of symptoms such as intermittent dizziness, incoordination, staggering, blurred vision, syncope, mental deterioration, and transient motor speech, or sensory deficits. These symptoms are often of such severity that daily activities may be markedly affected. The syndrome occurs frequently in connection with bilateral occlusion of the carotid while the collateral circulation functions satisfactorily.

Preoperative examination of such patients usually reveals multiple vascular occlusions and a global CBF that is considerably reduced. Tomographic findings show a moderate reduction of density in both hemispheres.

Although the superficial temporal artery can irrigate only a certain area of the hemisphere, increased flow in a certain region may nevertheless lead to an improvement in the general situation (Chater 1976). This can be explained by intracerebral and intracranial steal phenomena (Chapter 13). Although this syndrome has rarely been described in detail, there have been many references to it (Reichmann *et al.* 1975, Gratzl *et al.* 1976, Holbach *et al.* 1977). It is reported that patients with this syndrome who had undergone surgery experienced improved stimulation and general vitality, provided that the functioning of the anastomosis was satisfactory. Even those patients who needed constant care before the operation were able to look after themselves again, und bypass surgery can diminish the symptomatology dramatically (Chater *et al.* 1976). This improvement was also observed in one of our cases (case 29).

The generalized low-perfusion syndrome should be emphasized in the whole pattern of completed stroke, to which it also bears a clinical resemblance. Due to the generalized flow reduction, different problems exist in these cases, and we know from experience that a local flow increase may influence areas located farther away (Chapter 13).

13. Changes of Blood Flow Following Extra-Intracranial Bypass Procedure

Intra-arterial intraoperative blood pressure measurements by Yonekawa (1976) established that considerable flow and blood pressure is present in the superficial temporal artery equal almost to the systemic blood pressure. The pressure in the middle cerebral artery always proved to be 20 to 40 mm lower than in the superficial temporal artery. Sufficient flow to the cerebral area supplied by the middle cerebral artery was ensured by the higher pressure prevailing in the superficial temporal artery. The change of blood flow and pressure and sometimes the reversal of blood flow in vessels of the middle cerebral artery after an extra-intracranial anastomosis can certainly have repercussions on vascular areas some distance away, such as the anterior communicating artery and collateral circulations.

It is surprising that this fact is seldom mentioned in the literature, and then only incidentally. These "steal phenomena", as they generally appear in carotid artery occlusions, have been known for a long time and have also been found clinically, radiologically, and particularly in rCBF measurements by neurosurgeons dealing with extra-intracranial anastomosis. For example, in 1974 Austin described investigations of rCBF in 23 patients suffering from unilateral occlusions and stenoses. The CBF had dropped an average of 30 percent on the side of the lesion and 20 percent contralaterally. Similar results were reported by Schmiedek (1976).

From our data on 150 extra-intracranial anastomoses, we have chosen some typical cases in which a change of intracranial flow presumably took place postoperatively, or in which complications appeared that left no doubt that such changes had occurred.

Case Reports

Case 1: This 34-year-old woman was admitted to the hospital on February 2, 1975, after two TIA. Neurological examination revealed a hemiparesis on the right side. A four-vessel angiography showed a high-grade stenosis of the left internal carotid artery just proximal to the bifurcation (Figs. 91 and 92). On the basis of these findings, an extra-intracranial anastomosis on the left side was performed on February 5, 1975. No complications were observed postoperatively. Seven days after surgery the neurological symptoms had clearly improved. Ten days after the operation the patient again developed very mild transient hemiparesis which disappeared completely after several hours. Follow-up angiography 2 weeks after the operation showed a complete occlusion at the site where the stenosis had previously been. Blood flow in the area, usually supplied by the left middle cerebral artery, was ensured by a dilated superficial temporal artery (Figs. 93 and 94).

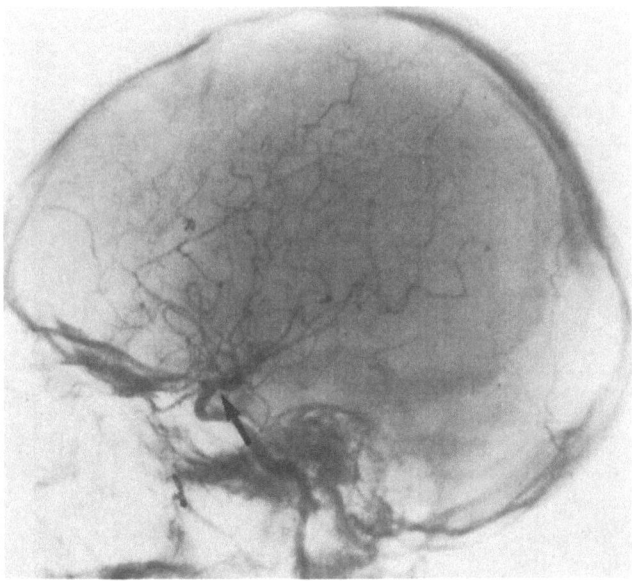

Fig. 91. Angiogram of the left internal carotid artery of a 34-year-old female with high-grade stenosis on the left internal carotid artery, just proximal to the bifurcation

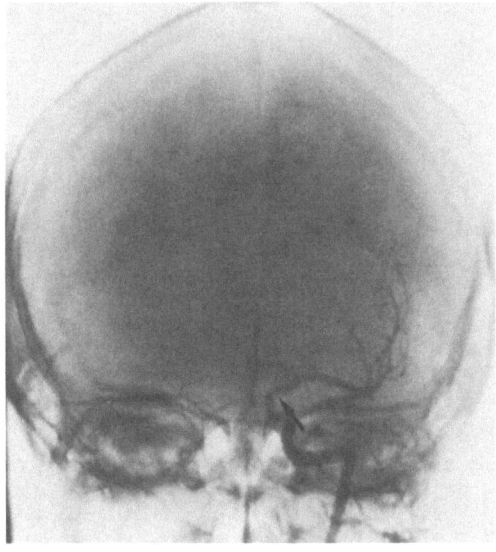

Fig. 92. Anteroposterior projection of angiogram shown in Fig. 91

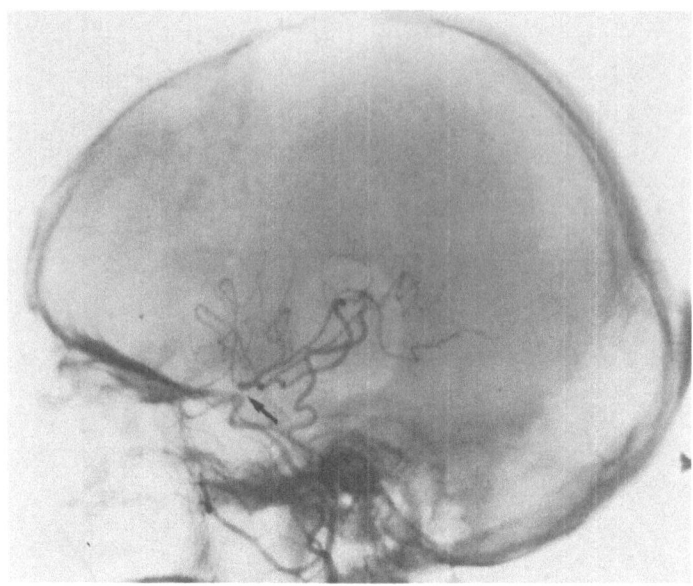

Fig. 93. Follow-up angiography 2 weeks after bypass operation in patient shown in Fig. 91 shows an occlusion in the region where the stenosis has been

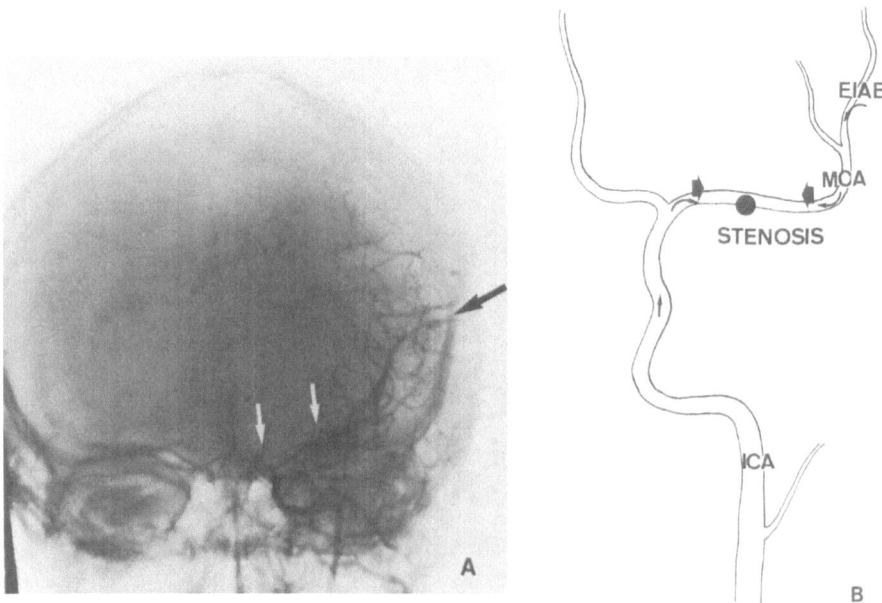

Fig. 94. Anteroposteriorprojection of angiogram shown in Fig. 93

There was no neurological deficit present when the patient was discharged from the hospital. No TIA have recurred on the right side during the past 4 years. In early 1976, one year after surgery, the patient was again admitted to the hospital after suffering two left-sided TIA. At the time of admission, there was no neurological deficit. A four-vessel angiography showed that the blood supply in the region of the left middle cerebral artery was well ensured by an enlarged superficial temporal artery. On the right side, there was a stenosis of the internal carotid artery slight exactly at the same site as on the left side 1 year before (Fig. 82 B, page 103). The patient refused to undergo another operation. She has been monitored continuously and had another two TIAs after her last hospitalization. Another follow-up angiography in early 1977 showed the same picture as in 1976: on the left side, good supply of the area of the middle cerebral artery via the anastomosis; on the right, stenosis in the middle cerebral artery. There was no change in the neurological status.

Comment

We believe it is quite conceivable that due to the left sided anastomosis the pressure gradient in the initial part of the middle cerebral artery or in the carotid artery was so low that when pressure was reversed, the stenosis rapidly turned into an occlusion (Fig. 94 B). We further believe that the short postoperative deterioration in the 10th postoperative day was the moment when occlusion in the left middle cerebral artery occurred. This theory is supported by the fact that the stenosis on the right side, where no surgery was performed, remained virtually unchanged, as confirmed by angiography after 1 year. In other words, no surgery was performed prior to occlusion of the left middle cerebral artery; this occlusion was provoked only by extra-intracranial anastomosis. We believe, however, that in this case surgery was indicated for the high-grade stenosis.

Case 2: This 42-year-old man was admitted after suffering a stroke accompanied by a considerable left hemiparesis. Four-vessel angiography showed a stenosis of the internal carotid artery in its siphon part on the right side (Fig. 95). On July 8, 1975, we performed an extra-intracranial anastomosis on the right side. Postoperatively, hemiparesis had clearly improved, so that after 3 months the patient was practically free of symptoms and could resume work (Fig. 96).

In connection with pneumonia, massive left paresis suddenly developed in this patient in December 1975, and he was again admitted to the hospital. Angiography now showed a complete occlusion of the internal carotid artery. The lenticulostriate arteries were affected. These two factors were the reason for the patient's severe neurological condition. The anastomosis itself was fully functioning, and the superficial temporal artery was dilated to more than twice its normal size (Fig. 97). However, only peripheral branches of the middle cerebral artery were supplied with blood by the anastomosis. The patient died 10 days after admission. Postmortem examination revealed extensive malacia of the right cerebral hemisphere; only the areas that had been supplied by the anastomosis were unaffected. The right internal carotid artery, the initial parts of the middle cerebral artery, and the anterior communicating artery were totally thrombosed.

Comment

In this patient, as in case 1, a stenosis obviously turned into an occlusion. Whether this was caused by the bypass itself, due to the changes pressure gradient (Fig. 97 B), or whether it was a result of progressive vascular disease cannot be stated with certainty.

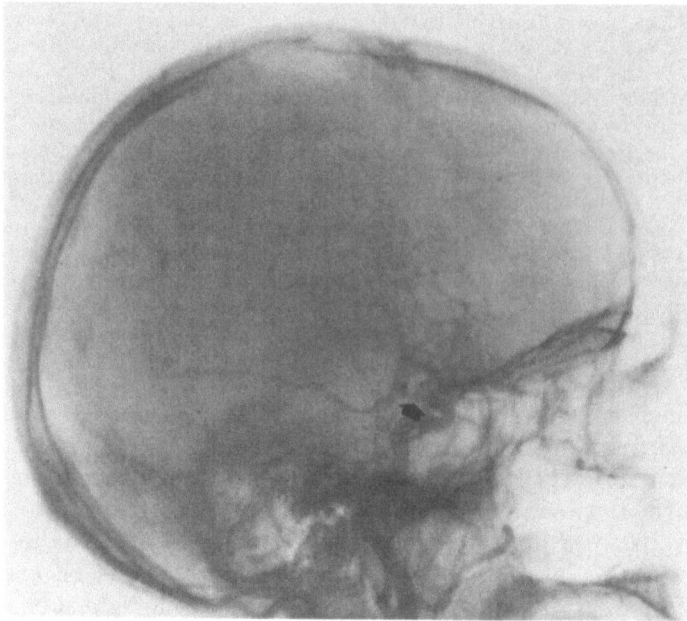

Fig. 95. A 42-year-old male with high-grade stenosis of the right internal carotid artery in the siphon

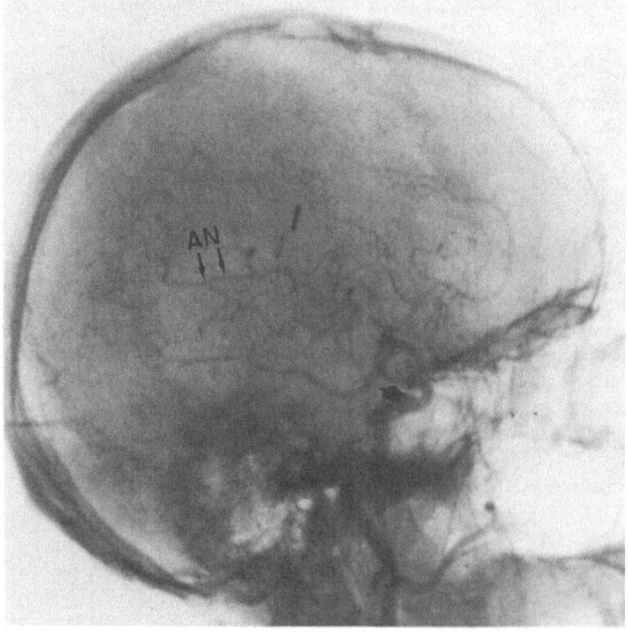

Fig. 96. Angiogram 14 days after operation in patient shown in Fig. 95. The anastomosis is working and the stenosis is visible

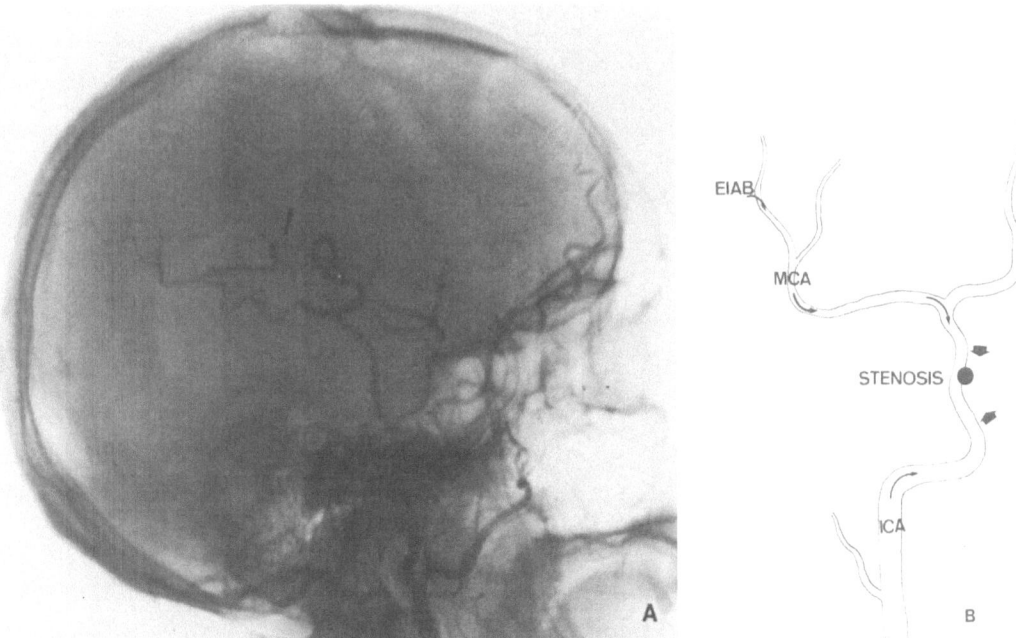

Fig. 97. Five months after the operation, the patient shown in Figs. 95 and 96 suddenly experienced deterioration and hemiparesis of the left side. The anastomosis was still working and the superficial temporal artery had enlarged, but there was complete occlusion of the carotid artery. The patient died 10 days later. The carotid artery and the middle cerebral artery were occluded by a large thrombus

Case 3: This 54-year-old man was admitted with a progressive stroke and three ischemic attacks. On admission, the patient was in a state of confusion; neurologically, medium-grade right hemiparesis was present. Four-vessel angiography showed a left carotid occlusion and stenosis of the right internal carotid artery in the siphon. The patient had a good cross flow through the anterior communicating artery from right to left, and there was sufficient collateral circulation through the ophthalmic artery on the left (Figs. 98, 99 and 100). Cerebral scintigraphy and computerized tomography showed a generalized reduction of blood flow with an ischemic focus on the left frontal side. rCBF measurement revealed reduced rates in both hemispheres; the CBF was lower by more than 30 percent on the side of the carotid occlusion. An extra-intracranial anastomosis was performed on the left side. There were no complications during the operation, and postoperatively the patient was well for a short time. One hour after the operation, there was a disturbance of consciousness and the patient suddenly developed high-grade left hemiparesis. Consequently a bilateral carotid angiography was conducted 24 hours after the operation, and it was found that the stenosis on the right side had developed into an occlusion. The anastomosis was patent. As far as collateral circulation was concerned, the left middle cerebral artery area was supplied by

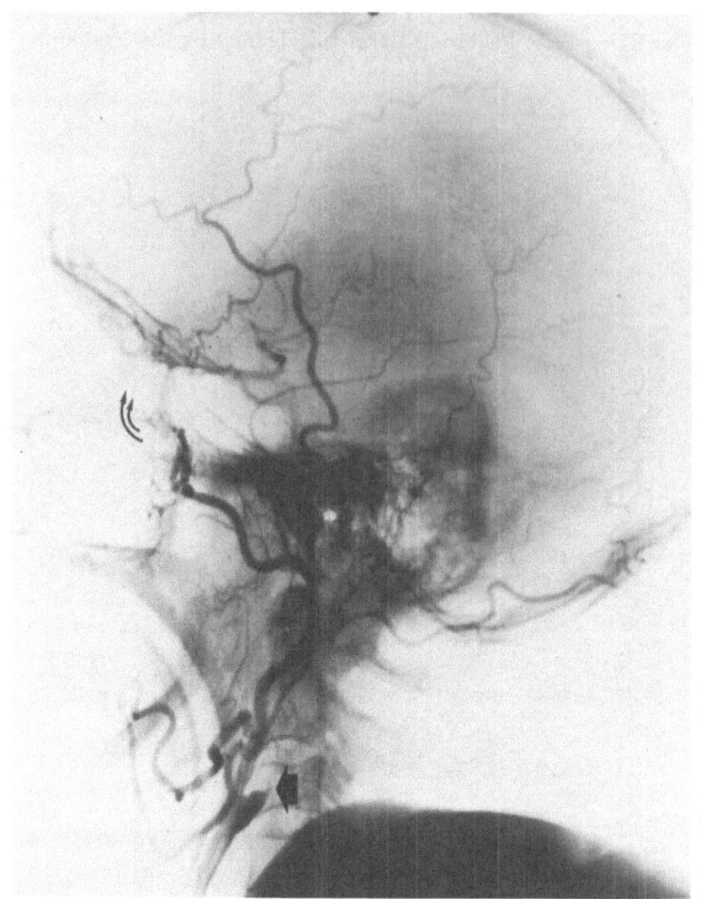

Fig. 98

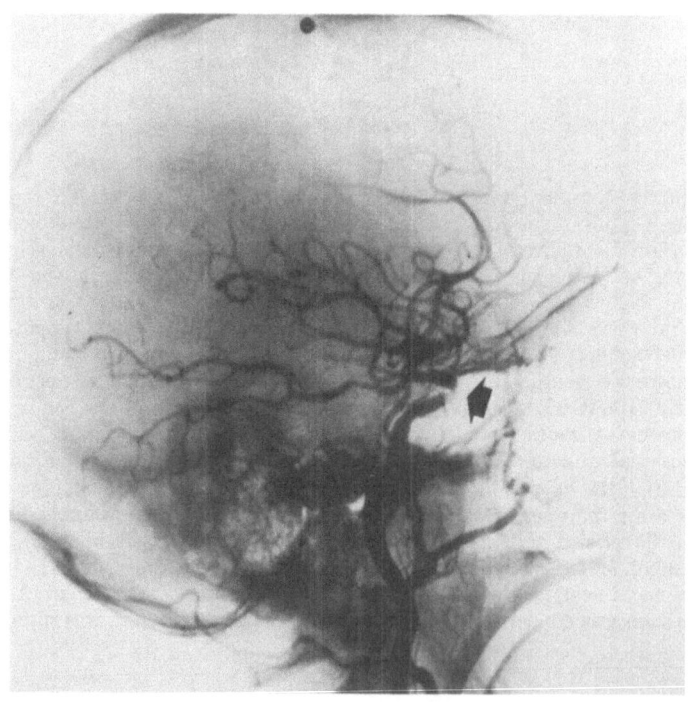

Fig. 99

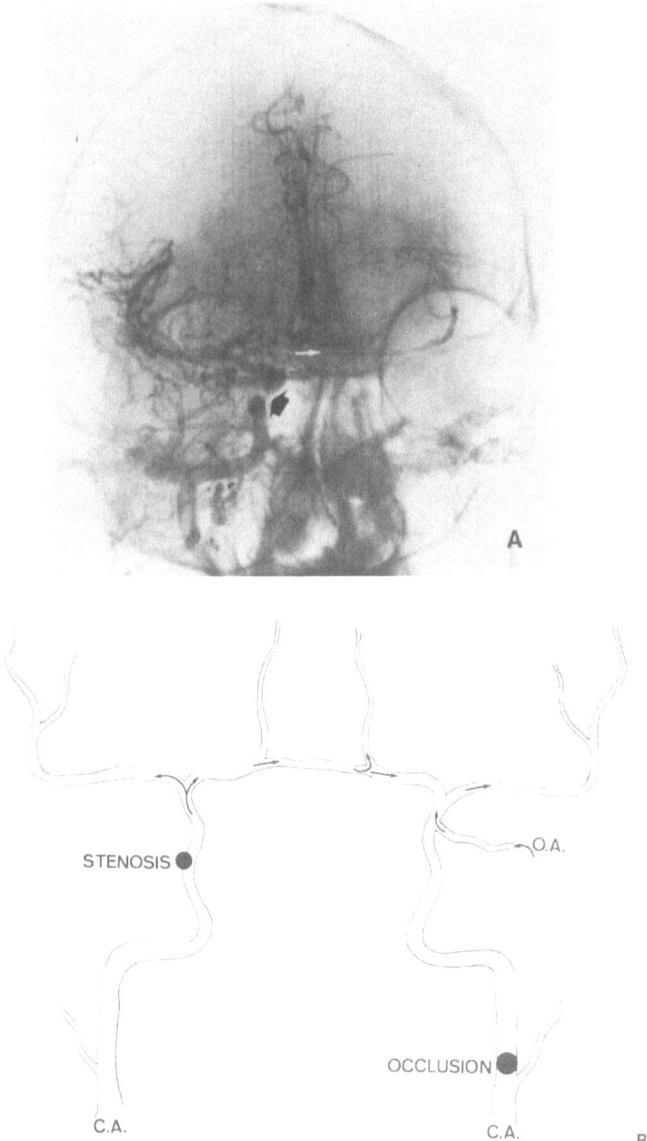

Fig. 100. Anteroposteriorprojection of angiogram shown in Fig. 99. Angiogram of the right carotid artery shows the stenosis in the siphon part of the carotid artery and sufficient collateral circulation via of the anterior cerebral artery to the middle cerebral artery on the left side

Fig. 98. Angiogram of the left carotid artery of a 54-year-old man with progressive stroke shows an occlusion of the internal carotid artery and very good collateral circulation through the ophthalmic artery on the left (↑↑)

Fig. 99. Angiogram of the right carotid artery of the patient shown in Fig. 98 shows a high-grade stenosis in the siphon

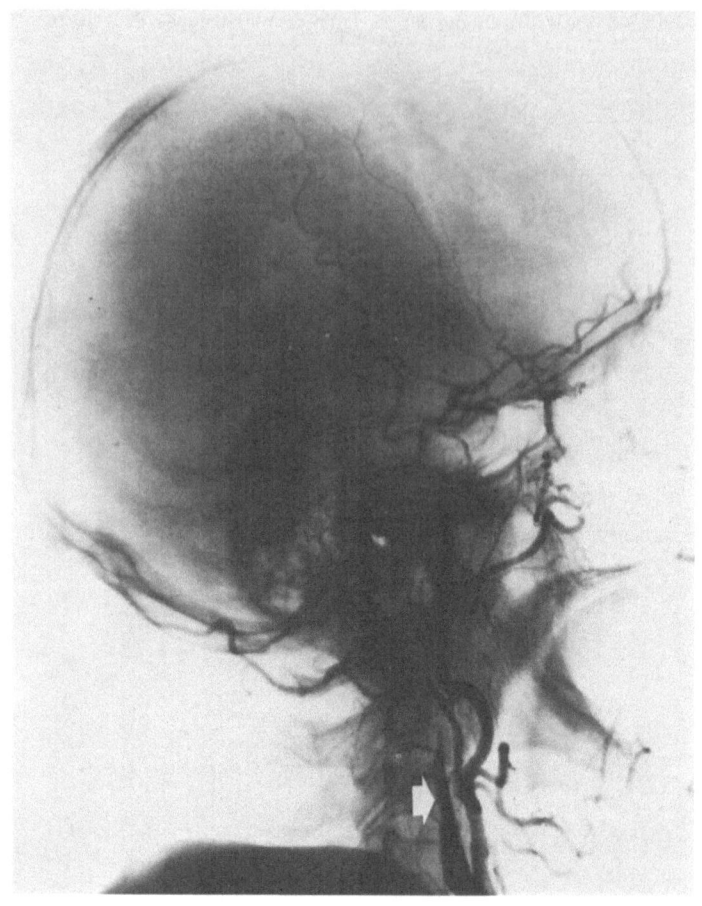

Fig. 101

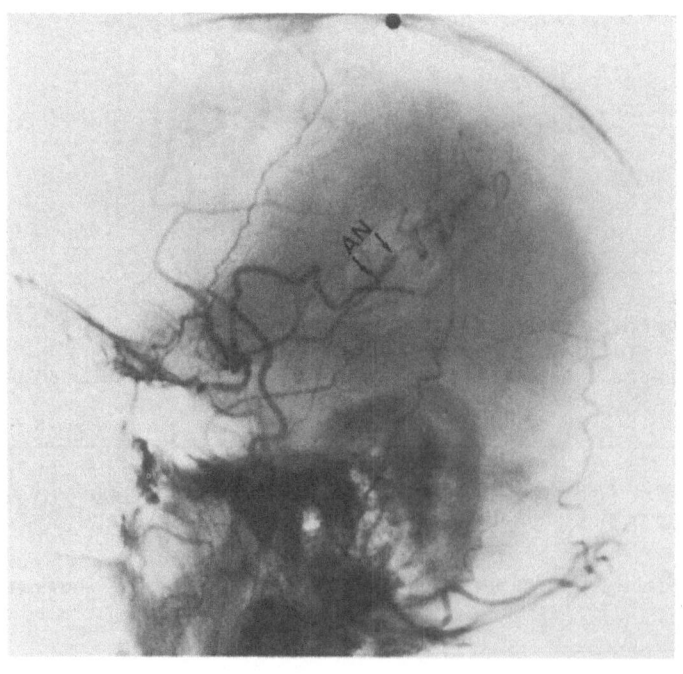

Fig. 102

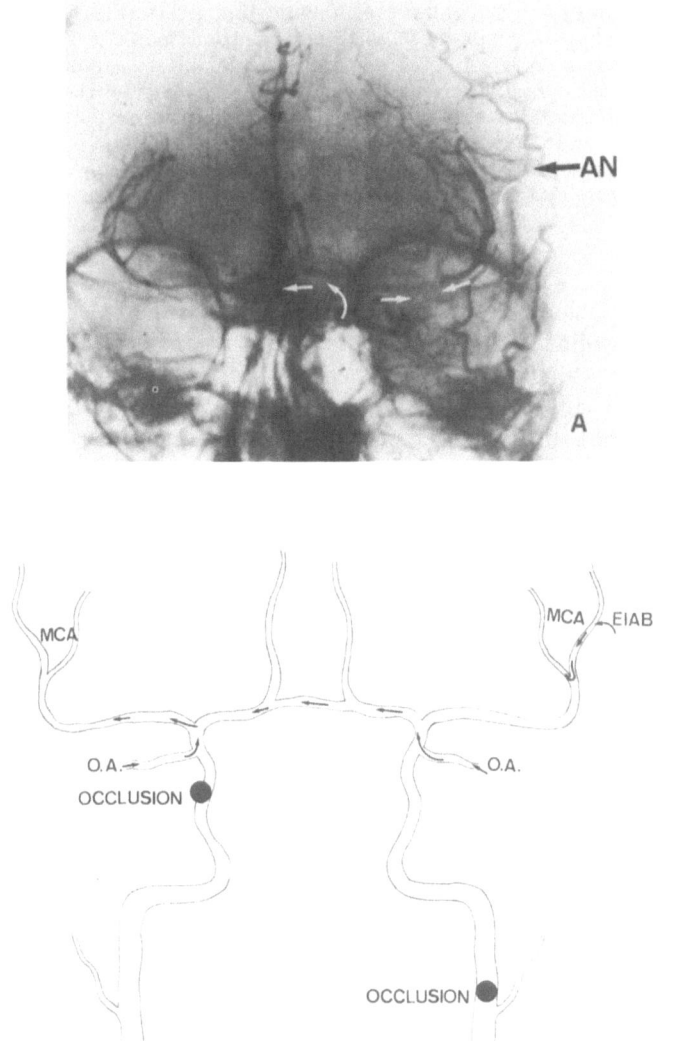

Fig. 103. Anteroposteriorprojection of angiogram shown in Fig. 102. Now an inversion of the blood flow from the left ophthalmic artery to the right middle cerebral artery is visible (see Fig. 100). The superficial temporal artery supplies the left region of the middle cerebral artery over the anastomosis

Fig. 101. Twenty-four hours after operation the condition of the patient shown in Figs. 98 through 100 was suddenly bad. The right carotid artery shows an occlusion and collateral circulation through the ophthalmic artery, now on the right side

Fig. 102. Angiogram of the left side of patient shown in Fig. 101 shows the anastomosis and good filling of the region of the middle cerebral artery on the left side

the functioning anastomosis, whereas the right cerebral hemisphere was supplied by the left ophtalmic artery and the anterior communicating artery (Figs. 101 to 103). These angiographic findings explain the clinical deterioration: namely, the left superficial temporal artery was not yet dilated and thus was unable to supply the left cerebral hemisphere, and the ophtalmic artery was not sufficient enough for the right hemisphere. A right sided extra-intracranial anastomosis was performed on the same day. It was impossible, however, to save the patient. His condition deteriorated progressively and he died on the 5th postoperative day. Postmortem findings were total malacia of the right cerebral hemisphere and partial malacia of the left hemisphere.

Comment

In this patient, extra-intracranial anastomosis combined with artificial new collaterals obviously provoked a complete breakdown of the previously established physiological collateral system. The pressure gradient in the right internal carotid artery apparently dropped to a very low level, so that the stenosis rapidly developed into a complete occlusion. The collateral circulatory system was not able to supply both hemispheres completely via the left superficial temporal artery and the left ophthalmic artery. It should also be noted that in this case a right-sided extra-intracranial anastomoses was probably not indicated because of the acute stroke.

Case 4: This 47-year-old patient had a left hemiparesis on admission to the hospital. Four-vessel angiography showed an occlusion of the right carotid, with a stenosis of the left internal carotid artery in its siphon part. The results of cerebral scintigraphy and computerized tomography were normal. rCBF measurement showed reduced blood flow in both hemispheres, with the right one more severely affected than the left. An extra-intracranial anastomosis was performed on the right side. The patient was initially very well; 12 hours after the operation, however, right hemiparesis developed suddenly. Follow-up angiography revealed a successful anastomosis on the right side, whereas the left internal carotid artery was now completely occluded. The patient recovered very rapidly from this postoperative incident and was discharged with a residual right paresis.

Comment

In this patient, the extra-intracranial anastomosis on the right side obviously changed the pressure gradient on the left internal carotid artery in its siphon part, so that it occluded. As in case 3, it is hardly inconceivable that a progressive disease became manifest just a few hours after the operation.

In 1974, Weinstein and Chater reported the case of a female patient operated on for high-grade stenosis of the middle cerebral artery. One year later, follow-up angiography showed a good blood supply to the cerebral hemisphere through the anastomosis. The stenosis of the middle cerebral artery had turned into an occlusion. It was assumed by the authors that this development, which is almost analogous to that in case 1 reported above, could be regarded as a progression of an underlying disease. This interpretation was supported by the fact that it took 1 year to complete the occlusion. However, it is not known at what time the stenosis turned into an occlusion. No other well-documented cases have been found in the literature. In a high-grade stenosis of the middle cerebral artery or the terminal part of the internal carotid artery near the bifurcation, it is conceivable that, due to hemodynamics, occlusion can be provoked by extra-intracranial bypass.

The problem of steal phenomena has already been mentioned. For example, in most of the patients suffering from unilateral carotid occlusion who Austin (1974) examined by means of rCBF measurement, both hemispheres showed reduced blood flow. This was also demonstrated by Schmiedek and Gratzl (1976). Apparently, a stenosed carotid siphon is a particularly vulnerable area. Yaşargil (1970) reported nine cases of extra-intracranial anastomoses. In two of these patients the anastomosis did not function or functioned only insufficiently postoperatively, and one patient presented a severe postoperative deterioration of neurological symptoms; both of these patients had a carotid stenosis in the siphon part. In Yaşargil's case 7, it was significant that while a left carotid occlusion existed prior to the operation there were symptoms originating primarily from the posterior cranial fossa. Postoperative angiography after deterioration of the patient's condition revealed an additional stenosis of the basilar artery, which had not been noticed before. In this case, too, it may be assumed that a change in flow also affected collaterals some distance away. The posterior cranial fossa was particularly affected.

In all the cases presented in this chapter, the anastomosis was on the side of the carotid occlusion, whereas the postoperative complications stemmed from a stenosis in the contralateral carotid artery. A similar case was reported by Chater in 1976. The surgical procedure involved the right side, with right carotid occlusion and left carotid stenosis. Chater reported that the patient's condition deteriorated acutely 5 days after the operation and that he finally died. The cause of the patient's death was concluded to be embolism induced by stenosis. This case study does not mention whether the patient underwent angiography after the operation or whether a postmortem examination was carried out. This case closely resembles cases 3 and 4 presented in this study.

On the other hand, several authors (Chater 1970, Deruty 1976, Holbach 1977) have described patients suffering from unilateral carotid occlusion and contralateral stenosis who showed very good postoperative results. In all of these patients the operation was performed on the side of the stenosis, since the symptoms originated from the stenosis. No postoperative angiography was reported in any of these cases. A high-grade stenosis can certainly occlude without causing significant symptoms, particularly if extra-intracranial anastomosis was performed ipsilaterally. This conclusion is supported by case 1 above.

Deruty (1974) reported two patients who were operated on the ipsilateral side of the stenosis. He wrote "that indication for surgery when carotid stenosis and carotid occlusion are simultaneously present is certainly a problem", without going into this problem any further.

Thus, when extra-intracranial anastomosis surgery is indicated in cases where a stenosis exists in the siphon, several factors have to be taken into account: first, the severity of the stenosis; and, second, whether the extra-intracranial bypass can supply such an area in the acute phase of occlusion. In the author's opinion, surgery should not be performed for a medium-grade stenosis. It should be treated only clinically, and in some cases it may be monitored radiologically. Surgery is really indicated only if a high-grade stenosis exists in the siphon.

These risks associated with extra-intracranial-bypass operation, which may affect more distant vascular regions in regard to blood flow and pressure, determine the procedure used in *unilateral carotid occlusion* and *contralateral carotid stenosis*. At the Department of Neurosurgery, Vienna, we now operate *first* on *the stenosed internal carotid artery* in the cervical region, with an intraluminar shunt. Approximately 10 days after the operation, the carotid occlusion is operated on. No serious complications have occurred when this procedure was used. We believe this is a relatively safe method of performing an arterial reconstruction on both hemispheres (Chapter 11.6.1.).

14. Postoperative Mortality and Morbidity

As can be expected with this surgical method, the surgical risk is relatively low. A major part of the operation consists of the anatomic preparation of the superficial temporal artery. Surgical intervention in this region does not severely affect the general condition of the patient. The craniotomy and the further extension of it does not cause any strain to the patient. The preparation of the cortical vessel and the anastomosis itself, the technically most difficult part of the operation, takes place in the cortex. Intervention in this region does not involve any risk either. It should be remembered, however, that the anesthesia itself represents a certain risk and that the patients involved in the operation frequently suffer from a severely damaged circulatory system. Although the actual operation is more or less harmless, a surgical risk is involved because the majority of patients have a general sclerotic disease, such as coronary arteriosclerosis, the aftereffects of myocardiac infarction, or stenoses of the large peripheral vessels. The mortality rate nonetheless must be considered to be very low. All major statistics report a surgical mortality rate (i. e., death occurring within 30 days after the operation) of between 3 and 5 percent.

Deaths that occur later than 4 weeks after operation cannot be attributed to the operation itself. In the available statistics the so-called late deaths also include numerous cardiac infarctions due to the basic disease. According to the author's own experience (Table 14), 50 percent of the late deaths must be attributed to cardiac infarction.

The late deaths should be classified with the cases of postoperative morbidity. The distinction to be made here is which hemisphere was involved in the new stroke—the one operated on or the other.

It must be emphasized that cerebrovascular disease associated with arteriosclerosis is a generalized affliction with progressive development. Improvement of the afflicted brain hemisphere is of primary concern. Since the sclerosis develops progressively, further attacks may occur later in the contralateral hemisphere.

Overall morbidity can also be influenced to a decisive extent since an extra-intracranial bypass can also have repercussions in the contralateral hemisphere (Chater 1976). The postoperative *morbidity rate* in TIA in Chater's study was 26 percent. In our study it slightly exceeded 20 percent. This means that the morbidity rate is reduced by two-thirds if one takes into account the fact that a 50 percent probability exists for TIA patients to have a manifest stroke within 1 year (Table 13, page 125).

According to the literature, 29 to 40 percent of patients with

Table 14. *Causes of Death After Extra-Intracranial Anastomosis (n = 150)*

Case No.	Early death (within 4 weeks after surgery)	Late death
1		cardiac infarction (34 months)
6		cerebral infarction (3 months)
7		cerebral infarction (7 months)
33	Astrozytome (3 weeks)	
44	Cerebral infarction (10 days)	
69		cardiac infarction (15 months)
74	Occlusion of aortic arch (3 weeks)	
76	Cerebral infarction (3 days)	
78	Cerebral infarction (5 days)	
101	Cerebral infarction (26 days)	

completed strokes die from another stroke within 3 years. In Gratzl's (1976) series of 29 operations in patients with completed stroke, there was only 1 death, and this was due to a glioblastoma.

In our series of 46 patients followed for more than 3 years after operation, 2 patients died of cerebral infarction 3 and 7 months after surgery (cases 6 and 7).

There is no question that the extra-intracranial bypass operation can influence the morbidity and mortality in stroke (Tables 12, 13, page 125). More exact data will only be obtained when a larger statistical sample exists after a period of approximately 20 years.

15. Considerations for the Future

Since the introduction of microvascular surgery, this technique has gained ground in the various medical disciplines. In neurosurgery, reconstructive vascular surgery is difficult because of the vulnerability of the central nervous system. Thus only extra-intracranial anastomosis has gained major importance. Perspectives, on the basis of this method, are as follows:

1. further improvement of preoperative diagnostic techniques so that an accurate indication for this operation can be determined,

2. refinement of the surgical technique itself,

3. application of this method in other central nervous system locations.

Methods of identifying indications for surgery will be improved and may be broadened only as soon as more comprehensive statistics extending over longer periods of time become available. This accumulation of data is being attempted at present by the "cooperative study" undertaken by Barnett and Peerless. Furthermore, the continued use of computerized tomography will probably provide more accurate indications for this surgical method.

The improvement of the surgical method must focus on the anastomosis itself with which possible mistakes affecting anastomosis function are associated. Moreover, this method is known to entail a lengthy operation, and the possibility of completing the operation, especially the anastomosis itself, within a shorter time would be advantageous.

15.1. Gluing of Microanastomoses

At the Department of Neurosurgery, Vienna, we have tried to perform microanastomosis by means of a new adhesive that does not affect the central nervous system. This was first accomplished in experiments and then clinically. The following questions had to be clarified for this purpose:

1. Is it possible to reduce the number of sutures needed when combining gluing and suturing, or is it even possible to do it completely without sutures?

2. Is gluing less traumatic for the vascular wall than suturing?

3. Is work easier and less time consuming if suturing and gluing are combined?

The experiments were carried out on the common carotid artery of 40 male Wistar rats (average weight: 250 g).

As gluing material we used a fibrinogen concentrate (Immuno-Wien) produced from human blood plasma, with an average of 110 mg coagulable material per 1 ml of solution. Before the operation the deep-frozen concentrate was slowly heated to body temperature. The highly viscous solution was applied in a quantity of 5 to 8 ml. By subsequently dripping on an equal amount of thrombin solution, the fibrinogen was caused to coagulate. The thrombin solution was composed of thrombin

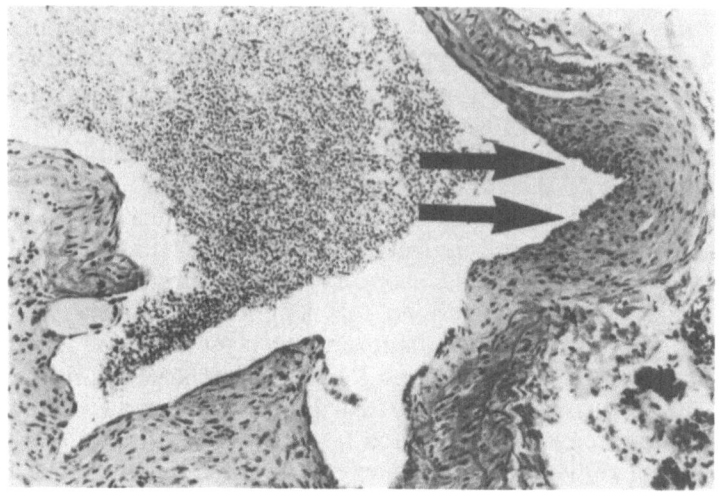

Fig. 104. Longitudinal section of end-to-end anastomosis 18 days after gluing. At the site of the welded anastomosis, the vascular wall is composed of a cicatricial tissue with tight fibers arranged in concentric lamellae (arrows). H + E. × 35

dissolved in 1 ml of Ringer's solution enriched with calcium ions (CaC_2 concentration: 5.46 mM/liter). The high thrombin concentration and the presence of calcium ions accelerated the clotting time to 4 to 6 seconds.

Under the operating microscope the common carotid artery of one side was laid bare. After proximal and distal clipping with microclamps, the vessel was cut transversely. Then two sutures were applied at 180 degrees. Next, first the front wall, and after turning the vessel, the back wall was glued by dripping fibrinogen concentrate and then thrombin solution on the vessel in a slightly everted position. Approximately 3 minutes after gluing, first the distal, then the proximal microclamp was opened and removed. The operating region was then closed with a suture.

The postoperative survival time for 30 animals was 2 to 21 days; for 10 animals it was 28 to 48 days. The efficiency of the anastomoses was sometimes checked by angiography, and in all cases by histological examination.

In sacrificed animals, the anastomosed vessels were exposed under the operating microscope, severed at a distance of at least 5 mm peripherally and centrally from the anastomosis, removed, and placed on a cork. After fixation in 5 percent neutral formalin, they were embedded in paraffin. Approximately seven longitudinal sections were made and stained with hematoxylin-eosin. A combined connective tissue and elastica stain, as well as Weigert's fibrin stain, were also used. These stains were performed only for animals surviving up to 7 days.

During the first 3 days after the operation, a fibrin cuff could be shown by means of Weigert's fibrin stain around the anastomosis. Under ideal conditions the everted vessel ends have approximately the same diameter as the arterial wall. During the first days, thromboses may adhere to the inner part of the anastomotic region. On the third day, the fibrin cuff is infiltrated by leukocytes and then replaced by young richly celled granulation tissue. After 6 to 8 days this cuff may be twice as large as the diameter of the artery without causing a narrowing of the arterial lumen. Around the sutures typical foreign body granulation tissue develops with the participation of giant cells. As the granulation tissue is rich in cells, in the course of the second week hyaline necroses appear to some extent around the suture material, which shows everted media parts.

At the end of the second postoperative week, the granulation tissue gives way to a cicatricial tissue with tight fibers rich in elastic lamellae that shows a concentric onion peel structure and has a diameter about twice as large as the vascular wall (Fig. 104).

Dehiscence in the anastomotic region is the most common complication, leading to a complete thrombotic occlusion of the vessel, which at a later date is often recanalized.

Of the 40 histologically examined anastomoses, 29 showed a patent narrow lumen. Three arteries were recanalized and 8 vessels either thrombosed or were obliterated by connective tissues.

Discussion

By combining gluing and suturing, only 2 sutures are necessary (instead of 8 to 12). These must be placed opposite each other so that the vessel ends fit exactly together. The key to successful gluing is the adaptation of the vessel ends. In the experimental setup we used, it is not possible to do completely without sutures. In the common carotid artery, a vessel rich in elastic membranes, the vessel stumps retract after severing, so that the adaptation sutures can be applied only under slight pressure. In gluing without sutures, the vessel ends should not be exposed to tension.

Most of the animals were kept alive up to 21 days after the operation. Histological examinations showed that the reparation process in the vascular wall was completed after 2 weeks. In cases of adaptational disorders accompanied by vascular thrombosis, recanalization of the obliterated vessel lumen can occur after a longer survival time. This makes long-term results questionable. If the vessel ends are exactly adapted, this type of gluing is an ideal method and considerably more physiological than suturing. Above all, fibrin gluing does not traumatize the vascular wall.

This method of surgery has also been applied in man. For 2 years the new adhesive has been used in all cases of extra-intracranial anastomosis. The time required to suture the anastomosis was thus reduced by 50 percent. The autopsy of a patient who died some time after the operation revealed that the anastomosis was much better from a histological point of view than might have been achieved with conventional suturing. This result corresponds to the histological study of the common carotid artery of the rat (Matras *et al.* 1976, Kletter *et al.* 1977, Meyermann *et al.* 1978).

15.2. Microanastomoses in the Spinal Cord Region

The application of the microvascular technique in other locations of the central nervous system presents a number of difficulties. Direct anastomoses on the basal cerebral arteries—for example, between two anterior cerebral arteries in the absence of a communicating artery, as was attempted by Yaşargil (1973)—is extremely difficult due to the location and the size of the vessels.

At the Department of Neurosurgery, Vienna, we have tried to apply the method of microvessel anastomosis on spinal vessels. Both in degenerative and traumatic spinal vasculopathies, surgery is generally confined to decompression of the spinal cord and operative interventions on the aorta and its branches. Recent experience in microvascular surgery, particularly in anastomosing small-caliber vessels with a patent diameter of no more than 0.6 mm, has paved the way for attampts at revascularizing the spinal cord by local microvascular procedures. A vascular approach appears to be well justified, since investigations by Tönnis (1953) and more recent studies indicated that slight to moderate trauma predominantly affected the blood supply of the spinal cord, while lesions of the spinal cord itself were only found to occur as a consequence of severe injuries. These findings prompted us to conduct the experiments reported here.

15.2.1. End-to-Side Anastomosis Between an Intercostal Artery Branch and a Dorsal Spinal Artery

Our initial experiments aimed at revascularizing the spinal cord by means of microvascular anastomoses in the thoracic spinal region. Sheep and dogs appeared to be well suited as experimental animals for this purpose since their vascular system and spinal canal structure are comparable to those of humans.

A branch of the intercostal artery was chosen as the afferent vessel. In the area of the autochthonous dorsal muscles this is the only vessel that shows a relatively constant course and is present in each thoracic segment. In addition, it courses in the immediate vicinity of the spinal canal. Consequently, dissection of the vessel can be limited to a length of 5 to

6 cm. End-to-side anastomosis was attempted after laminectomy and the selection of a suitable spinal vessel. As expected, anastomosis proved to be quite problematic since the diameter of arterial vessels in this area is usually between 0.4 and 0.6 mm.

The technique was employed in 5 sheep and 10 dogs. Due to the small size of the vessels, satisfactory anastomoses were obtainable in only 9 cases. In 6 of these, appreciable hemorrhagic malacia and edema of the spinal cord developed in the anastomosed area after removal of the clip from the afferent vessel. In one case the anastomosis performed well originally, but 24 hours after surgery a complete hemiplegic syndrome developed and the animal had to be sacrificed. Histologically, there was again appreciable hemorrhagic malacia. In 2 cases we saw no postoperative changes.

15.2.2. Pedicled Muscle Grafting Onto the Spinal Cord

There have been many successful attempts at revascularizing ischemic structures with the help of pedicled muscle grafts. In 1944 Henschen convincingly demonstrated the revascularization of ischemic brain areas by temporal muscle transplants. The concept was later adopted in cardiac surgery (Blalog 1951), and in 1974 Yaşargil et al. showed that in dog brains the transplantation of abundantly vascularized tissues, such as the omentum and muscle tissue, produced an ingrowth of blood vessels into the central nervous system if it was meticulously adapted to neural structures.

To our knowledge, there have been no attempts at transplanting muscle tissue onto the spinal cord thus far, although the autochthonous muscles in this area appear to be ideally suited for this purpose.

At the thoracic level selected for the experiment, a longitudinal skin incision was made. This was continued laterally, curving along the costal arch at an obtuse angle. The skin flap thus obtained can readily be reflected cranially so that both muscles and spinal cord can be seen. Laminectomy was performed in the usual way. The muscle was then detached from its fascia and part of it was dissected cranially with a pedicle caudally. After incision of the dura, the muscle graft was pressed onto the spinal cord and adapted. This technique was used in 10 dogs and 10 rats. In 3 dogs, paraplegic symptoms developed immediately after surgery. Since these symptoms failed to improve, the animals were sacrified 6 hours after surgery.

This complication can be expointed for by a faulty technique: either the muscle tissue implanted intradurally was excessively thick, with resultant dural compression, or dural sutures overlying the muscle graft were excessively tight. In the remaining 7 dogs no neurologic deficits whatever were observed. The animals were sacrificed after 3 months. The histological examination showed noticeable ingrowth of small vessels into the spinal cord.

Of the 10 rats treated, 1 showed paraplegic symptoms immediately after surgery. It was kept alive, however, for another week, since nursing proved to be unproblematic. Subsequently, 2 animals were sacrificed at intervals of 1 week, thus the histological developments were recorded over a period of 5 weeks. As in the nonsymptomatic dogs, there was evidence of an ingrowth of small capillaries into the spinal cord (Fig. 105).

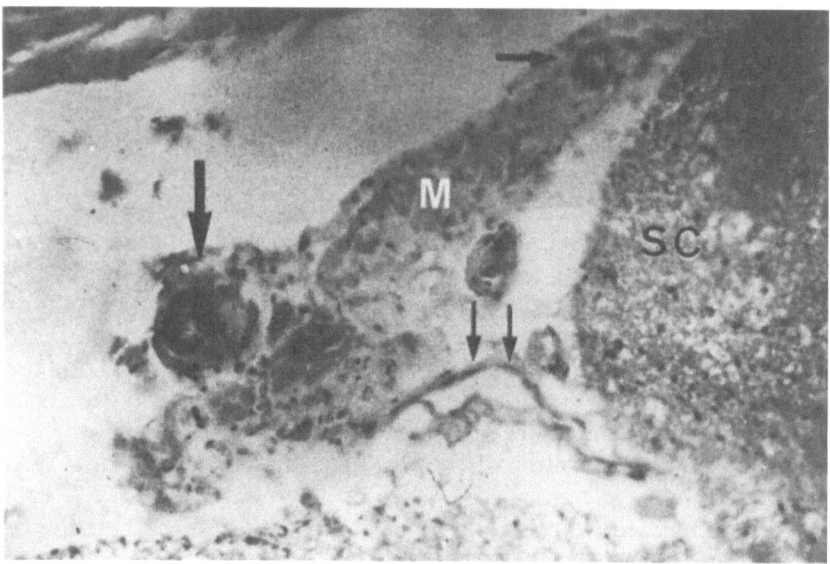

Fig. 105. Histological examination of transplantation of muscle to the spinal cord 3 months after operation. A transverse section of the spinal cord is shown. Small vessels (double arrows) from the muscle (*M*) are in connection with the spinal cord (*SC*). Single arrow: arteries of the muscle. H + E × 60

Discussion

In diseases and traumatic lesions of spinal cord vessels both conservative and surgical treatment have made hardly any appreciable advances in recent decades. As microsurgical techniques have become more sophisticated in recent years, delicate structures, particularly small-caliber vessels, have become accessible to surgery. Microvascular surgery, however, has failed to produce truly satisfactory microvascular anastomoses in the spinal area. While microanastomoses of vessels with a caliber down to 0.6 mm have repeatedly been shown to be functional (Piza-Katzer 1974), they have invariably been attempted in regions that are less susceptible to hypoxia than the spinal cord. Problems encountered in attempts at a direct local anastomosis of spinal vessels include the following:

1. Extremely small caliber of the vessels to be anastomosed (0.4 to 0.6 mm),

2. Clipping time,

3. Flow direction at the anastomosis site (potential steal effect),

4. Inadequate venous drainage (venous anastomosis).

Microanastomoses of vessels in the caliber range of 0.4 to 0.6 mm are technically possible, provided that a suitable technique is used and that the surgeon has sufficient experience. Clipping time appears to be a crucial problem. We believe it to be the primary factor underlying the development of malacia, which was present in virtually all cases treated.

While these two problems may be eliminated, the direction of blood flow continues to be a problem, since a reverse flow may produce a steal effect above or below the anastomosis with resultant undesirable hypoxemia in another segment.

Venous drainage is, in our view, the cardinal factor. Experience in transplantation surgery had repeatedly shown that an increased blood flow through an arterial anastomosis is poorly tolerated by damaged tissue as long as venous drainage is inadequate. Consequently, we believe that for spinal microanastomoses to function properly both arterial and venous anastomoses are required. Although a venous pathway would theoretically be available for anastomosis in the vicinity of the artery described, the technique we used was inadequate for producing a venous anastomosis in the caliber range encountered in this area.

We have found the transplantation of a pedicled muscle flap to be the more promising technique for a successful revascularization of the spinal cord. In virtually all cases treated, a more or less extensive ingrowth of small capillaries from the adjacent muscle was found to occur into the central nervous system. Nevertheless, there are still some unsolved problems; the timing of surgery on what is essentially damaged tissue is one of them. Long-term effects are as yet unknown.

We hope that this work may encourage further investigation along these lines.

References

Abercrombie, J.: Über die Krankheiten des Gehirns und des Rückenmarks. Bonn: Weber. 1821.

Acheson, J., Hutchinson, E. C.: Observations on the natural history of transient cerebral ischemia. Lancet *11* (1964), 871—874.

Acland, R.: Signs of patency in small vessel anastomosis. Surgery *72* (1972), 744—748.

— Prevention of thrombosis in microvascular surgery by the use of magnesium sulfate. Brit. J. Plast. Surg. *25* (1972), 292—304.

Ahlgren, P.: Moyamoya disease: bilateral occlusion of the carotid artery associated with abnormal vascular network in the basal region of the brain. Dan. Med. Bull. *23* (1976), 41—45.

Ainsworth, R. W., Gresham, G. A., Balmforth, G. V.: Pathological changes in temporal arteries removed from unselected cadavers. J. Clin. Path. *14* (1961), 115—119.

Allcock, J. M.: Occlusion of the middle cerebral artery. Serial angiography as a guide to conservative therapy. J. Neurosurg. *27* (1967), 353—363.

Amine, A. R. C., Moody, R. A., Meeks, W.: Bilateral temporal-middle cerebral artery anastomosis for moyamoya syndrome. Surg. Neurol. *8* (1977). 3 6.

Anderson, R. E., Reichman, O. H., Davis, D. O.: Radiological evaluation of temporal artery—middle cerebral artery anastomosis. Radiology *113* (1974), 73—79.

Arnold, S. L.: Carotid endarterectomy: a perspective. South Med. J. *69* (1976), 896—898.

Auld, A. W.: Transient ischemic attacks not produced by extracranial vascular disease: a plea for complete and early angiographic investigation. South Med. J. *69* (1976), 722—724.

Ausman, J. I., et al.: Stroke: What's new? Cerebral revascularization. Minn. Med. *59* (1976), 223—227.

Austin, G. (ed.): Microsurgical anastomoses for cerebral ischemia. Springfield, Ill.: Ch. C Thomas. 1976.

Austin, G., Laffin, D., Hayward, W.: Indications and results of micro bypass surgery for cerebral ischemia. Second International Symposium on Microneurosurgical Anastomoses for Cerebral Ischemia. Chicago, Illinois (1974).

——— Physiologic factors in the selection of patients for superficial temporal artery—to—middle cerebral artery anastomosis. Surgery *75* (1974), 861—868.

——— Microcerebral anastomosis for the prevention of stroke. In: Handa, H. (ed.): Microneurosurgery, pp. 47—67, Tokyo: Igaku Shoin. 1975.

——— Cerebral blood flow and pressure in patients undergoing STA-MC anastomosis. Second International Symposium on Microneurosurgical Anastomoses for Cerebral Ischemia. Chicago, Illinois (1974).

Bailey, J. C., Kiryabwire, J. W. M.: Traumatic aneurysms of the superficial temporal artery. Brit. J. Surg. *60* (1973), 530—532.

Baker, R. N., Ramseyer, J. C., Schwartz, W. S.: Prognosis in patients with transient cerebral ischemic attacks. Neurology (Minneap.) *18* (1968), 1157—1165.

Bannister, C.: Anastomosis of small vessels in growing animals. Proceedings of the First International Symposium on Microneurosurgical Anastomoses for Cerebral Ischemia. Loma Linda, California (1973).

Baxter, Th. J., O'Brien, B., Menderson, P. N., Bennet, R. C.: Die Histopathologie der Vernarbung an kleinen Gefäßen. Brit. J. Surg. *59* (1972), 617—621.

Beevor, C. E.: The cerebral artery supply. Brain *30* (1907), 403—425.

Berguer, R., et al.: Vertebral artery bypass. Arch. Surg. *111* (1976), 976—979.

Bone, G. E., et al.: Clinical implications of the Doppler cerebrovascular examination: a correlation with angiography. Stroke 7 (1976), 271—274.

Bone, G. E., Barnes, R. W.: Limitations of the Doppler cerebrovascular examination in hemispheric cerebral ischemia. Surgery 79 (1976), 577—580.

Bossi, R., Piasini, C.: Collateral cerebral circulation through the ophthalmic artery and its efficiency in internal carotid occlusions. Brit. J. Radiol. 28 (1955), 462—469.

Bret, P., Dechaume, J. P., Deruty, R.: Traitement chirurgical des embolies artérielles intracrâniennes. Lyon Med. 229 (1973), 679—691.

Brenner, H., Zaunbauer, W.: Über Fehlermöglichkeiten bei der zerebralen Angiographie. Radiol. Austr. 16 (1966), 45—52.

Brenner, H., Kletter, G.: Diagnostik und Therapie des Carotisverschlusses. Neurol. Diagnostik 1978.

Buncke, H. J., Schultz, W. P.: Experimental digital amputation and reimplantation. Plast. Reconstr. Surg. 36 (1965), 62—71.

Burrows, E. H., Marshall, J.: Angiographic investigations of patients with transient ischemic attacks. J. Neurol. Neurosurg. Psychiat. 28 (1965), 533—539.

Butzer, J. F., et al.: Transient ischemic attacks. Compr. Ther. 1 (1975), 31—35.

Carney, A. L.: Ocular plethysmography. Second International Symposium on Microneurosurgical Anastomoses for Cerebral Ischemia. Chicago, Illinois (1974).

Carpenter, M. B., Noback, C. R., Moss, M. L.: The anterior choroidal artery. Its origins, course, distribution and variations. Arch. Neurol. Psychiat. 71 (1954), 714—722.

Chater, N. L., Spetzler, R., Mani, J.: The spectrum of cerebrovascular occlusive disease suitable for microvascular bypass surgery. Angiology 26 (1975), 235—251.

Chater, N. L.: Anatomic localization of optimal middle cerebral branch for STA anastomosis. First International Symposium on Microneurosurgical Anastomoses for Cerebral Ischemia. Loma Linda, California (1973).

— Patient selection and results of extra- to intracranial anastomosis in selected cases of cerebrovascular disease. Clin. Neurosurg. 23 (1976), 287—309.

— Surgical results and measurements of intraoperative flow in microneurosurgical anastomoses. In: Austin, G. M. (ed.): Microneurosurgical anastomoses for cerebral ischemia, pp. 295—304. Springfield, Ill.: Ch. C Thomas. 1976.

Chater, N. L., Peerless, S. J., Weinstein, Ph. R.: Review of experiences with 50 consecutive cases of superficial temporal to middle cerebral artery anastomosis for treatment of cerebrovascular occlusive disease. Second International Symposium on Microneurosurgical Anastomoses for Cerebral Ischemia. Chicago, Illinois (1974).

Chater, N. L., Weinstein, P., Peters, N.: Neurosurgical microvascular bypass for stroke. Meeting of the American College of Surgeons, San Francisco, October 1975.

Chater, N. L., Spetzler, R., Tonnemacher, K., Wilson, Ch.: Microvascular bypass surgery. Part I: Anatomical Studies. J. Neurosurg. 44 (1976), 712—714.

Chater, N. L., Popp, J.: Microsurgical vascular bypass for occlusive cerebrovascular disease: review of 100 cases. Surg. Neurol. 6 (1976), 115—118.

Chater, N. L., Mani, J., Tonnemacher, K.: Superficial temporal artery bypass in occlusive cerebral vascular disease. Calif. Med. 119 (1973), 9—13.

Chiari, H.: Über das Verhalten des Teilungswinkels der Carotis communis bei der Endarteriitis chronica deformans. Verh. Dtsch. Ges. Pathol. 9 (1905), 326—330.

Chou, S. N.: Embolectomy of middle cerebral artery. Report of a case. J. Neurosurg. 20 (1963), 161—163.

Cobbett, J. R.: Microvascular surgery. Surg. Clin. N. Amer. 47 (1967), 521—524.

Cohnheim, W.: Untersuchungen über die embolischen Prozesse. Berlin: A. Hirschwald. 1872.

Collaborative Group for the Study of Stroke in Young Women: Oral contraception and increased risk of cerebral ischemia or thrombosis. New Engl. J. Med. 288 (1973), 871—878.

Conant, R. G., Perkins, J. A., Ainley, A. B.: Stroke morbidity, mortality and rehabilitative potential. J. Chron. Dis. 18 (1965), 397—423.

Conforti, P., Cioffi, F. A., Tomasello, F., Albanese, V.: Review of microneurosurgical anastomosis for cerebral ischemia. Second International Symposium on Microneurosurgical Anastomoses for Cerebral Ischemia. Chicago, Illinois (1974).

Corbett, J. L.: Hypertension and strokes. Drugs *11*, Suppl. 1 (1976), 27—34.

Corkill, G., French, B. N., Michas, C., Cobb, C. A., Mims, T. J.: External carotid-vertebral artery anastomosis for vertebrobasilar insufficiency. Surg. Neurol. *7* (1977), 109—115.

Cormier, J. M.: Surgical management of vertebral-basilar insufficiency. J. Cardiovasc. Surg. (Torino) *17* (1876), 205—223.

— Surgical management of vertebral-basilar insufficiency. Int. Surg. *61* (1976), 203—212.

Crow, R. L.: Treatment of evolving strokes. J. Arkansas Med. Soc. *72* (1976), 323—326.

Crowell, R. M.: Electromagnetic flow studies of superficial temporal artery to middle cerebral branch artery bypass graft. In: Austin, G. M. (ed.): Microneurosurgical anastomoses for cerebral ischemia, pp. 116—124. Springfield, Ill.: Ch. C Thomas. 1976.

Crowell, R. M., Olsson, Y.: Effects of extracranial-intracranial vascular bypass graft on experimental acute stroke in dogs. J. Neurosurg. *38* (1973), 26—31.

Crowell, R. M., Yaşargil, M. G.: End-to-side anastomosis of superficial temporal artery to middle cerebral artery branch in the dog. Neurochirurgia *16* (1973), 73—77.

Cusick, J. F., Komacki, S., Choi, H.: Superficial temporal-middle cerebral artery anastomosis associated with glioblastoma multiforme. Case report. J. Neurosurg. *46* (1977), 381—384.

Danzinger, J.: The pathological basilar artery. Clin. Radiol. *27* (1976), 309—316.

Davis, D. O.: Use to computerized tomography in stroke. Second International Symposium on Microneurosurgical Anastomoses for Cerebral Ischemia. Chicago, Illinois (1974).

De Bakey, M. E.: Concepts underlying surgical treatment of cerebrovascular insufficiency. Clin. Neurosurg. *10* (1964), 310—340.

De Bakey, M. E., Crawford, E. S., Cooley, D. A., Morris, G. C., Garrett, H. E., Fields, W. S.: Cerebral arterial insufficiency: one to 11-year results following arterial reconstructive operation. Ann. Surg. *161* (1965), 921—932.

De Long, W. B.: Anatomy of the middle cerebral artery: The temporal branches. Stroke *4* (1973), 412—418.

Deruty, R., Lecuire, J., Bret, P., Dechaume, J. P., Lapras, C.: Tentatives de revascularisation cérébrale par l'anastomose extra-intracrânienne dans certaines ischémies. Neuro-chirurgie (Paris) *20* (1974), 345—368.

Deruty, R., Duquesnel, J., Lecuire, J., Dechaume, J. P., Bret, P.: L'anastomose extra-intracrânienne; corrélations radio-cliniques. Neuro-chirurgie (Paris) *22* (1976), 469—476.

Deruty, R.: Experimental studies preparing for human extra-intracranial anastomosis. In: Austin, G. M. (ed.): Microneurosurgical anastomoses for cerebral ischemia, pp. 125—132. Springfield, Ill.: Ch. C Thomas. 1976.

Donaghy, R. M. P., Yaşargil, M. G.: Microanginal surgery and its techniques. Progr. Brain Res. *30* (1968), 263—267.

Donaghy, R. M. P.: Evaluation of extracranial-intracranial blood flow diversion. In: Austin, G. M. (ed.) Microneurosurgical anastomoses for cerebral ischemia, pp. 256—274. Springfield, Ill.: Ch. C Thomas. 1976.

Donaghy, R. M. P., Yaşargil, M. G.: Extra-intracranial blood flow diversion. American Association of Neurological Surgeons. Chicago, Illinois, April 11 (1968).

—— Micro-vascular surgery. St. Louis: The C. V. Mosby Co., G. Thieme. 1967.

Donaghy, R. M. P.: What's new in surgery. Neurologic surgery. Surg. Gynec. Obstet. *134* (1972), 269—272.

Dorndorf, W.: Gegenwärtiger Stand der chirurgischen Behandlung des zerebrovaskulären Insults. Nervenarzt *36* (1965), 18—30.

— Verlauf und Prognose bei spontanen zerebralen Arterienverschlüssen. Heidelberg: Dr. A. Hüthig. 1968.

— Verlauf und Prognose des ischämischen Hirninfarktes. Nervenarzt *40* (1969), 297—302.

Driesen, W.: Erfolgreiche Naht der linken Arteria Cerebri Media nach Verletzung durch Tumorresektion. Acta Neurochir. (Wien) *10* (1962), 462—465.

Dujovny, M., Osgood, P. C., Maroon, J. C.: Canine cerebral ischemia: A preliminary model to evaluate microvascular anastomoses. Second International Symposium on Microneurosurgical Anastomoses for Cerebral Ischemia. Chicago, Illinois (1974).

Dujovny, M., Osgood, C. P., Barrionuevo, P.: Experimental middle cerebral artery microsurgical embolectomy. Acta Neurochir. (Wien) *35* (1976), 91—96.

———— Middle cerebral artery microneurosurgical embolectomy. Surgery *80* (1976), 336—339.

Eastcott, M. H. G., Pickering, G. W., Robb, C. G.: Reconstruction of internal carotid artery in a patient with intermittant attacks of hemiplegia. Lancet *2* (1954), 994—996.

Egli, H., Regli, F., Baumgartner, G.: Die Prognose des Karotisverschlusses und der Karotisstenose mit abgeschlossenem zerebralem Insult unter konservativer und nach operativer Therapie. Schweiz. Arch. Neurol. Neurochirurg. Psychiatr. *111* (1972), 243—257.

Ehringer, H.: Thrombolytische Therapie bei Durchblutungsstörungen. Öst. Ärzteztg. *30/5* (1975), 281—287.

Einsiedel-Lechtape, H.: Arteriosclerosis of the brain vessels as an indication to vascular surgery. I. Neurosurg. Sci. *19* (1975), 23—28.

Ekeströms: Ischemic cerebrovascular lesions (4). Surgical treatment. Lakartidningen *73* (1976), 3979—3984.

Epstein, M. H.: Anastomosis of saphenous vein graft to cortical branches of the middle cerebral artery. Second International Symposium on Microneurosurgical Anastomoses for Cerebral Ischemia. Chicago, Illinois (1974).

Evans, R. B., Austin, G.: Psychological evaluation of patients undergoing microneurosurgical anastomoses for cerebral ischemia. In: Austin, G. M. (ed.): Microneurosurgical anastomoses for cerebral ischemia, pp. 320—326. Springfield, Ill.: Ch. C Thomas. 1976.

Fazio, C.: Autoregulation des Hirnkreislaufes. Triangel *9* (1970), 244—249.

Fein, J. M., Molinari, G.: Experimental augmentation of regional blood flow by microvascular anastomosis. J. Neurosurg. *41* (1974), 421—426.

Fein, J. M., Reichman, O. H. (eds.): Microvascular anastomoses for cerebral ischemia. Berlin-Heidelberg-New York: Springer. 1978.

Ferguson, G. G., Drake, C. G., Peerless, S. J.: Extracranial-intracranial arterial bypass in the treatment of "giant" intracranial aneurysms. Stroke *8* (1977), 11.

Ferguson, G. G., Peerless, S. J.: Extracranial-intracranial arterial bypass in the treatment of dementia and multiple extracranial arterial occlusion. Stroke *7* (1976), 13.

Fields, W. S.: Selection of stroke patients for arterial reconstructive surgery. Amer. J. Surg. *125* (1973), 527—529.

Fields, W. S., Bell, R. M., Campbell, J. M.: Computered tomography in the management of cerebrovascular disease. Stroke *6* (1975), 105—107.

Fields, W. S., North, R. R., Hass, W. K., Galbraith, J. G., Wylie, J. E., Ratinov, G., Burns, H. M., MacDonald, M. C., Meyer, J. S.: Joint study of extracranial arterial occlusion as a cause of stroke. Jama *203* (1968), 955—960.

Fine, R. D.: Treatment of cerebrovascular disease. Curr. Ther. *17* (1976), 39—48.

Fisher, M.: Occlusion of the internal carotid artery. Arch. Neurol. Psych. *65* (1951), 346—377.

Fitzgerald, D. E., Horris, L. E.: Temporal arteriitis: A review of some current literature. Canad. mes. Assoc. J. *84* (1961), 108—112.

Fraser, R. A.: The role of surgery in ischemic stroke. Postgrad. Med. *59* (1976), 135—139.

Friedman, G. D., Wilson, W. S., Mosier, J. M., Colandrea, M. A., Nichaman, M. Z.: Transient ischemic attacks in a community. Jama *210* (1969), 1428—1434.

Gänshirt, H.: Der Hirnkreislauf. Stuttgart: G. Thieme. 1972.

Galibert, P., Delcour, J., Grunewald, P., Petit, P., Rosat, P.: Oblitérations de l'artère sylvienne. Traitement chirurgical ou médical. Neuro-chirurgie (Paris) *17* (1971), 165—176.

Garrido, E.: Middle cerebral artery embolectomy. Case report. J. Neurosurg. *44* (1976), 517—521.

Gillilan, L. A.: Potential collateral circulation to the human cerebral cortex. Neurology *24* (1974), 941—948.

Goldberg, H. I.: Recent advances in cerebral angiographic examination of stroke. In: Salomon, G., Advances in cerebral angiography, pp. 208—215. Berlin-Heidelberg-New York: Springer. 1975.

Gordon, E. E., Kohn, K. H.: Evaluation of rehabilitation methods in the hemiplegic patient. J. Chron. Dis. *19* (1966), 3—16.

Gratzl, O., Schmiedek, P., Spetzler, R., Steinhoff, H., Marguth, F.: Clinical experience with extra-intracranial arterial anastomosis in 65 cases. J. Neurosurg. *44* (1976), 313—324.

Gratzl, O., Schmiedek, P.: Microneurosurgical arterial anastomosis in patients with prolonged reversible ischemic neurological deficits (PRIND). Second International Symposium on Microneurosurgical Anastomoses for Cerebral Ischemia. Chicago, Illinois (1974).

Gratzl, O., Schmiedek, P., Steinhoff, H., Enzenbach, R.: The significance of regional cerebral blood flow (rCBF) studies for microvascular surgery in patients with cerebral ischemia. Second International Symposium on Microneurosurgical Anastomoses for Cerebral Ischemia. Chicago, Illinois (1974).

Gratzl, O., Schmiedek, P., Steinhoff, H.: Extra-intracranial arterial bypass in patients with occlusion of cerebral arteries due to trauma and tumor. In: Handa, J. (ed.): Microneurosurgery. Tokyo: Igaku Shoin. 1975.

Gratzl, O., Steude, U., Schmiedek, D.: Indications for extra-intracranial anastomosis between the superficial temporal artery and a branch of the middle cerebral artery in man. In: Fusek, J., Kunce, Z.: Present Limits of Neurosurgery, pp. 375—379. Amsterdam: Excerpta Medica. 1972.

Gratzl, O., Schmiedek, P., Steinhoff, H., Enzenbach, R.: Quantitative and regional effects of microneurosurgical anastomosis in patients with cerebral ischemia. Europ. Surg. Res. *6* (1974), 27.

Gratzl, O., Schmiedek, P., Steinhoff, H.: Five year follow-up of 65 patients treated with extra-intracranial arterial bypass for cerebral ischemia. In: Advances in Neurosurgery, Vol. 3, pp. 115—117. Berlin-Heidelberg-New York: Springer. 1976.

Gratzl, O.: Microneurosurgical anastomoses for cerebral ischemia in 39 patients—clinical results, angiography and regional cerebral blood flow. In: Austin, G. M. (ed.): Microneurosurgical anastomoses for cerebral ischemia, pp. 308—319. Springfield, Ill.: Ch. C Thomas. 1976.

— Neurosurgical therapy of inadequate cerebral circulation. Internist *17* (1976), 38—44.

Gregorius, F. K., Rand, R. W.: Scanning electron microscopic observations of common carotid artery endothelium in the rat. Surg. Neurol. *4* (1975), 258—264.

Gros, Q., Minvielle, J., Vlahovitch, B.: Anastomoses artérielles intracrâniennes. Etude artériographique et clinique. Neuro-chirurgie (Paris) *2*, 3 (1956), 281—302.

Gutrecht, J. A.: Occult temporal arteriitis. Jama *213* (1970), 1188—1189.

Guthrie, C. C.: Blood vessel surgery and its application, pp. 222—293. London: E. Arnold. 1912.

— Some physiologic aspects of blood-vessel surgery. Jama *51* (1908), 1658—1667.

Haas, W. K., Fields, W. S., North, R. R., Kricheff, J. J., Chase, N. E., Baurer, R. B.: Joint study of extracranial arterial occlusion. Arteriography, techniques, sites and complications. Jama *203* (1968), 961—968.

Handa, J., Handa H.: Progressive cerebral arterial occlusive disease: analysis of 27 cases. Neuroradiol. *3* (1972), 119—133.

Hartl, O., Pürgyi, P.: Risikofaktoren für den cerebralen Insult. Prakt. Arzt *29* (1975), 270—281.

Heilbrun, M. P., Reichman, O. H., Anderson, R. E., Roberts, Th. S., Powell, Ch. B.: Regional CBF studies following superficial temporal-middle cerebral artery anastomosis. Second International Symposium on Microneurosurgical Anastomoses for Cerebral Ischemia. Chicago, Illinois (1974).

Heilbrun, M. P., Reichman, O. H., Anderson, R. E., Roberts, Th. S.: Regional cerebral blood flow studies following superficial temporal-middle cerebral artery anastomosis. J. Neurosurg. *43* (1975), 706—716.

Henschen, C.: Operative Revascularisation des zirkulatorisch geschädigten Gehirns durch Auflage gestielter Muskellappen. (Encephalo-Myo-Synangiose). Langenbecks Arch. Chir. *264* (1950), 392—401.

Herrschaft, M.: Die quantitative Messung der örtlichen Hirndurchblutung. Ihre Bedeutung für die Diagnostik und Therapie der cerebralen Durchblutungsstörungen. Frankfurt/Main 1972.

Herman, L. H., Ostrowski, A. Z., Gurdjian, E. S.: Perforating branches of the middle cerebral artery: An anatomical study. Arch. Neurol. (Chicago) *8* (1963), 32—34.

Hoedt-Rasmussen, K., Sveinsdottir, E., Lassen, N. A.: Regional blood flow in man determined by intraarterial injection of radioactive inert gas. Circ. Res. *18* (1966), 237—247.

Hoedt-Rasmussen, K.: Regional cerebral blood flow. The intraarterial injection method. Copenhagen: Munksgaard. 1967.

Holbach, K. H., Wassmann, H., Bodosi, M., Bonatelli, A. P.: Superficial temporal-middle cerebral artery anastomosis for internal carotid occlusion. Acta Neurochir. (Wien) *37* (1977), 201—217.

Hollin, S. A., Silverstein, A.: Transient occlusion of the middle cerebral artery. Jama *194* (1965), 243—247.

Hollin, S. A., Sukoff, M. H., Silverstein, A., Gross, S. W.: Posttraumatic middle cerebral artery occlusion. J. Neurosurg. *25* (1966), 526—535.

Hossman, K. A., Sato, K.: Recovery of neuronal function after prolonged cerebral ischemia. Science (1970), 168—375.

Hounsfield, G. N.: Computerized transverse axial scanning (tomography). I. Description of system. Brit. J. Radiol. *46* (1973), 1016—1024.

Inaba, Y., Komatsu, K., Fukushima, Y.: Small arterial replacement with tefron graft—an experimental study. In: Handa, J. (ed.): Microneurosurgery, p. 18. Tokyo: Igaku Shoin. 1975.

Ingvar, D. H., Cronquist, S., Ekberg, R., Risberg, J., Hoedt-Rasmussen, K.: Normal values of regional cerebral blood flow in man, including flow and weight estimates of grey and white matter. Acta Neurol. Scand. Suppl. *14* (1965), 72.

Ingvar, D. H., Risberg, J.: Increase of regional cerebral blood flow during mental effort in normals and in patients with focal brain disorders. Exp. Brain Res. *3* (1967), 195—211.

Ingvar, D. H.: Regional cerebral blood flow in cerebrovascular disorders. Progr. Brain Res. *30* (1968), 57—61.

Irino, T., Taneda, M., Minahi, T.: Angiographic manifestations in postrecanalized cerebral infarction. Neurology *27* (1977), 471—475.

Ito, Z., Hen, R., Nakajima, K., Onuma, T., Moriyama, T.: Indications for surgical treatments and selections of operative procedures in occlusive cerebrovascular diseases. Surgery *38* (1976), 352—361.

Ito, Z., Hen, R., Nakajima, K., Suzuki, A., Moriyamat, T., Nemura, K.: Evaluation of functional reversibility of ischemic brain—to select appropriate patients with completed stroke for STA-MCA bypass surgery. Neurologia Medico-Chirurgica *16* (1976), 121—129.

Isler, W.: Akute Hemiplegien und Hemisyndrome im Kindesalter. Stuttgart: Thieme. 1969.

Jacobson, J. H., Wallman, L. J., Schumacher, G. A., Flanagan, M., Suarez, E. L., Donaghy, R. M. P.: Microsurgery as an aid to middle cerebral artery endarterectomy. J. Neurosurg. *19* (1962), 108—114.

Jacobson, J. H., Suarez, E.: Microsurgery in anastomosis of small vessels. Surg. Forum *11* (1960), 243—245.

Jennett, W. B., Harper, M. A.: Measurement of regional cerebral blood flow during carotid ligation. Lancet *11* (1960), 1162—1167.

Keller, H., Baumgartner, G.: Doppler-Ultrasonographie: Eine nicht belastende Untersuchungsmethode zur Diagnose und Therapiekontrolle von Karotisstenosen. Schweiz. Med. Wschr. *104* (1974), 1281—1291.

Kety, S. S., Schmidt, C. F.: The nitrous oxide method for the quantitative determination of cerebral blood flow in man: Theory, procedure, and normal values. J. Clin. Invest. *27* (1948a), 476—483.

— — The effects of altered arterial tensions of carbon dioxide and oxygen on cerebral blood flow and cerebral oxygen consumption of normal young men. J. Clin. Invest. *27* (1948), 484—491.

Khodadad, G.: Middle cerebral artery embolectomy and prolonged widespread vasospasm. Stroke *4* (1973), 446—450.

— Sublingual and lingual-basilar artery anastomoses and carotid-basilar bypass grafts. Surg. Neurol. *1* (1973), 175—177.

— Transient occlusion of temporal-middle cerebral anastomosis: Spasm, swelling or thrombosis. Surg. Neurol. *3* (1975), 341—375.

— Occipital artery-posterior inferior cerebellar artery anastomosis. Surg. Neurol. *5* (1976), 225—227.

— The superficial temporal artery-middle cerebral artery branch anastomosis. In: Austin, G. M. (ed.): Microneurosurgical anastomoses for cerebral ischemia, pp. 202—213. Springfield, Ill.: Ch. C Thomas. 1976.

Khodadad, G., Singh, R. S., Olinger, C. P.: Prevention of brain stem stroke by microvascular anastomosis in the vertebro-basilar system. Stroke *8* (1977), 11.

Kikuchi, H., Karasawa, J.: StA-Cortical MCA anastomosis for cerebrovascular occlusive disease. Neurol. Surg. (Tokyo) *1* (1973), 15—19.

— — Experience with STA-MC anastomoses on cerebral occlusion. Second International Symposium on Microneurosurgical Anastomoses for Cerebral Ischemia. Chicago, Illinois (1974).

— — Extra-intracranial arterial anastomosis in 9 patients with moya-moya disease. In: Schmiedek, P. (ed.): Microsurgery for Stroke. Berlin-Heidelberg-New York: Springer. 1977.

Kletter, G.: Tödliche Thrombosen bei Frauen im gebärfähigen Alter. Münch. Med. Wschr. *22* (1973), 1017—1019.

Kletter, G., Koos, W. Th.: Zur Technik der arteriellen experimentellen extra-intrakraniellen Anastomose. Acta Chir. Austriaca *7* (1975), 83—86.

Kletter, G., Feigl, W., Sinzinger, H.: Arteriosclerotic alterations of the superficial temporal artery in severe general sclerosis. In: Advances in Neurosurgery, Vol. 2, pp. 395—400. Berlin-Heidelberg-New York: Springer. 1975.

Kletter, G., Meyermann, R., Koos, W. Th., Schuster, H.: L'importance de la structure histologique de l'artère temporale superficielle pour la fonction de l'anastomose artérielle extra-intra-crânienne. Neuro-chirurgie (Paris) *21* (1975), 551—556.

Kletter, G.: The selection of cerebral arteries for extra-intracranial bypass. In: Koos, W. Th., Böck, F. W., Spetzler, R. F. (eds.): Clinical microneurosurgery. Stuttgart: Thieme. 1976.

Kletter, G., Feigl, W., Sinzinger, H.: The applicability of the superficial temporal artery for extra-intracranial bypass. In: Koos, W. Th., Böck, F. W., Spetzler, R. F. (eds.): Clinical microneurosurgery, p. 239. Stuttgart: Thieme. 1976.

Kletter, G., Meyermann, R.: Histological case control of microanastomoses. In: Koos, W. Th., Böck, F. W., Spetzler, R. F. (eds.): Clinical microneurosurgery, p. 234. Stuttgart: Thieme. 1976.

Kletter, G., Grunert, V.: Deutung und Mißdeutung problematischer Karotisangiogramme. Acta Chir. Austriaca, Suppl. 1976/77, 521—524.

Kletter, G., Meyermann, R.: Histologische Veränderungen nach Mikrogefäßanastomosen. Acta Chir. Austriaca *2* (1977), 35—38.

Kletter, G., Koos, W., Schuster, H.: Zur chirurgischen Therapie von Verschlüssen und Stenosen im Bereich der A. cerebri media. Kongreßbericht d. Österr. Ges. f. Chir. 18. Tagung/Graz, 19.—21. 5. 1977, S. 234—238.

Kletter, G., Meyermann, R., Grunert, V., Witzmann, A.: Beitrag zur rekonstruktiven Gefäßchirurgie des Rückenmarks. Acta Chir. Austriaca *3* (1977), 58—61.

Kletter, G., Meyermann, R., Ammerer, H. P., Witzmann, A.: Reconstructive surgery of spinal cord vessels. An experimental study. In: Advances in Neurosurgery, Vol. 4, pp. 327—329. Berlin-Heidelberg-New York: Springer. 1977.

Kletter, G., Meyermann, R., Witzmann, A.: Potential of reconstructive vascular surgery in the spinal cord—an experimental study. In: Schmiedek, P. (ed.): Microsurgery for Stroke, pp. 163—165. Berlin-Heidelberg-New York: Springer. 1977.

Kletter, G., Meyermann, R., Feigl, W., Sinzinger, H.: Importance of the histologic structure of the superficial temporal artery for the function of extra-intracranial bypass. In: Schmiedek, P. (ed.): Microsurgery for Stroke, pp. 139—141. Berlin-Heidelberg-New York: Springer. 1977.

Kletter, G., Matras, H., Dinges, H. P.: Zur partiellen Klebung von Mikrogefäßanastomosen im intrakraniellen Bereich. Wien. klin. Wschr. *90* (1978), 415—419.

Koos, W. Th., Böck, P., Spetzler, R. F.: Clinical microneurosurgery. Stuttgart: Thieme. 1976.

Koos, W. Th., Reichmann, O. H., Schuster, H., Kletter, G.: Surgical technique of extra-intracranial arterial anastomosis. In: Koos, W. Th., Böck, F. W., Spetzler, R. F. (eds.): Clinical microneurosurgery, p. 247. Stuttgart: Thieme. 1976.

Koos, W., Kletter, G., Schuster, H.: Probleme der extra-intracraniellen Gefäßanastomosen. Acta Chir. Austriaca, Suppl. 1976/77, 270—274.

Krayenbühl, H., Yaşargil, M. G.: Verschluß der A. cerebralis media, Ergebnisse der klinischen und katamnestischen Untersuchungen. Schweizer Arch. Neurol. Neurochir. Psych. *94* (1964), 287—296.

—— Die neuroradiologische Diagnostik und die chirurgische Therapie der Hirngefäßverschlüsse. Therapeut. Umschau *25* (1968), 462—469.

—— Die cerebrale Angiographie. Stuttgart: Thieme. 1965.

—— Der cerebrale kollaterale Blutkreislauf im angiographischen Bild. Acta Neurochir. (Wien) *6* (1958), 30—80.

Krayenbühl, H. A.: The Moyamoya syndrome and the neurosurgeon. Surg. Neurol. *4* (1975), 353—360.

Kudo, T.: Spontaneous occlusion of the circle of Willis: a disease apparently confined to Japanese. Neurology *18* (1968), 485—496.

Kurtzke, J. F.: Epidemiology of cerebrovascular disease. Berlin-Heidelberg-New York: Springer. 1969.

Lassen, N. A., Hoedt-Rasmussen, K., Sørensen, S. C. Skinhøj, E., Cronquist, S., Bodforss, B., Ingvar, D. H.: Regional cerebral blood flow in man determined by Krypton 85. Neurology *13* (1963), 719—727.

Lassen, N. A.: Cerebral blood flow and oxygen consumption in man. Physiol. Rev. *39* (1959), 183—187.

Lassen, N. A., Ingvar, D. H.: Regional cerebral blood flow measurement in man. A Review. Arch. Neurol. *9* (1963), 615—622.

—— The blood flow of the cerebral cortex determined by radioactive Krypton 85. Experientia (Basel) *17* (1961), 42—43.

Lazar, M. L., Clark, K.: Microsurgical cerebral revascularisation: concepts and practice. Surg. Neurol. *1* (1973), 355—359.

Lazorthes, G., Geraud, J., Bes, A.: Hämodynamische Untersuchungen und Pathologie der Hirngefäße. Triangel *9* (1970), 250—257.

Lecuire, J., Goutelle, A., Sray, G., Dechaume, J. P.: Indications thérapeutiques dans les thromboses traumatiques de l'artère carotide interne. Neuro-chirurgie (Paris) *11* (1965), 295—302.

Lecuire, J., Deruty, R., Bret, Ph., Dechaume, J. P., Yasui, H.: Anastomosis between superficial temporal artery and a branch of the middle cerebral artery (Abstract). In: Handa, J. (ed.): Microneurosurgery, pp. 82—83. Tokyo: Igaku Shoin. 1975.

Leeds, N. E., Abbott, K. H.: Collateral circulation in childhood via rete mirabile and perforating branches of anterior choroidal and posterior cerebral arteries. Radiology *85* (1965), 628—634.

Lie, J. T., Brown, A. L., Carter, E. T.: Spectrum of aging changes in temporal arteries. Arch. Path. *90* (1970), 278—285.

Lindgren, S. O.: Course and prognosis in spontaneous occlusions of cerebral arteries. Acta psychiat. neurol. Scand. *33* (1958), 343—354.

Little, J. R., Sundt, T. M., Kerr, F. H.: Neuronal alteration in developing cortical infarction. J. Neurosurg. *39* (1974), 186—198.

Lougheed, W. M., Elgie, R. G., Barnett, H. J. M.: The results of surgical management of extracranial internal carotid artery occlusion and stenosis. Canad. med. Ass. J. *95* (1966), 1279—1293.

Lougheed, W. M., Marshall, B. M., Hunter, M., Michel, E. R., Sandwith-Smith, M.: Common carotid to intracranial internal carotid bypass venous graft. J. Neurosurg. *34* (1971), 114—118.

Lougheed, W. M., Gunton, R. W., Barnett, H. J. M.: Embolectomy of internal carotid, middle and anterior cerebral arteries. J. Neurosurg. *22* (1965), 607—612.

——— Embolectomy of internal carotid, middle and anterior cerebral arteries. Report of a case. J. Neurosurg. *20* (1963), 161—163.

Mallett, B. L., Veall, N.: The measurement of regional cerebral clearance rates in man using 133 Xe inhalation and extracranial recording. Science *29* (1965), 179—184.

Maroon, J. C., Roberts, E., Numoto, M., Donaghy, P.: Microvascular surgery: simplified instrumentation. J. Neurosurg. *38* (1973), 119—124.

Maroon, J. C., Donaghy, D.: Experimental cerebral revascularization with autogenous grafts. J. Neurosurg. *38* (1973), 172—179.

Maroon, J. C.: Current concepts in cerebral revascularization with bypass grafts. In: Austin, G. M. (ed.): Microneurosurgical anastomoses for cerebral ischemia, pp. 35—38. Springfield, Ill.: Ch. C Thomas. 1976.

Marshall, J.: Angiography in the investigation of ischemic episodes in the territory of the internal carotid artery. Lancet *1* (1971), 719—721.

— The natural history of transient ischemic cerebro-vascular attacks. Quart. J. Med. *33* (1964), 309—324.

Mastri, A. R., Silverstein, P. H., Gold, L., Eselius, E. P.: Multiple progressive intracranial arterial occlusions. Stroke *4* (1973), 380—386.

Matras, H., Chiari, F. M., Kletter, G., Dinges, H. P.: Neue Wege in der Mikrogefäßchirurgie. Acta Chir. Austriaca, Suppl. 1976/77, S. 458—460.

——— Zur Klebung von Mikrogefäßanastomosen. (Eine experimentelle Studie.) 13. Jahrestagung d. Deutsch. Ges. f. Plast. u. Wiederherstellungschirurgie, Sept. 1975, Stuttgart, S. 357—360. Stuttgart: Thieme. 1976.

——— Zur Klebung kleinster Gefäße im Tierversuch. Dtsch. Z. Mund-Kiefer-Gesichts-Chir. *1* (1977), 19—23.

Matsubara, T.: Anastomosis of the middle cerebral artery with the external carotid branch for middle cerebral occlusion: application of microsurgery. Brain Nerve (Tokyo) *21* (1969), 645—650.

McHenry, L. C., Fazekas, J. F., Sullivan, J. F.: Cerebral hemodynamics of syncope. Amer. J. Med. Sci. *241* (1961), 173—177.

Melamed, E., Cahane, E., Carmon, A., Lavy, S.: Stroke in Jerusalem district 1960 through 1967: An epidemiological study. Stroke *4* (1973), 465—471.

Mennonna, P., Cagnoni, G.: Traumatic occlusion of the middle cerebral artery. J. Neurosurg. Sci. *21* (1977), 71—77.

Merei, F. T., Bodosi, M., Gallyas, F.: Über die Rolle der Fluoreszenzangiographie bei der Untersuchung und Behandlung der Kreislaufstörungen im Carotisgebiet. Ideggyogy. Szle. (hung) (1976).

Merei, F. T.: Reconstructive surgery of brain arteries. Budapest: Akadémiai Kiadó. 1976.

Merei, F. T., Bodosi, M.: Microsurgical anastomosis for cerebral ischemia in ninety patients. In: Schmiedek, P. (ed.): Microsurgery for Stroke. Berlin-Heidelberg-New York: Springer. 1977.

Meyermann, R., Kletter, G.: Ultrastructural findings after microsurgical interventions on the carotid artery of the rat. Acta Neurochir. (Wien) *35* (1976), 71—83.

Meyermann, R., Kletter, G., Koos, W. Th.: Morphologic changes after vascular microanastomoses as a function of the technique used. In: Schmiedek, P. (ed.): Microsurgery for Stroke, pp. 123—127. Berlin-Heidelberg-New York: Springer. 1977.

Meyermann, R., Wismann, H., Kletter, G.: Morphometric approach to fine structural changes in the intima of the common carotid artery of the rat following microsurgery. In: Schmiedek, P. (ed.): Microsurgery for Stroke. Berlin-Heidelberg-New York: Springer. 1977.

——— Morphologische Veränderungen an kleinen Gefäßen nach mikrochirurgischen Eingriffen. In press.

Meyermann, R., Kletter, G., Wismann, H.: Die Ultrastruktur der A. carotis communis der Ratte nach renaler Hypertonie. In press.

Meyermann, R., Kletter, G., Budka, H.: Die Histologie extra-intrakranieller Anastomosen zur Behandlung cerebraler Ischämien. In press.

Miller, J. D., Stanek, A. E., Langfitt, Th. W.: Cerebral blood flow regulation during experimental brain compression. J. Neurosurg. 39 (1973), 186—196.

Mintschev, D.: Electroencephalographic findings in vertebrobasilar circulation disorders. Psychiat. Neurol. med. Psychol. (Leipzig) 27 (1975), 470—476.

Moran, J. M., Reichman, O. H., Baker, W. H.: Staged intracranial and extracranial revascularization. Arch. Surg. 112 (1977), 1424—1428.

Mosmans, P. C. M.: Regional cerebral blood flow in neurological patients: Clinical significance and correlation with E.E.G. Van Gorcum: Assen. 1974.

Neblett, R.: Pontage entre la carotide cervical et la carotide interne intracrânienne à l'aide de technique de micro-chirurgie vasculaire. In: L'ischémie cérébrale dans le territoire carotidien. Rev. Méd. Toulouse 9 (1973), 447—449.

Newman, M.: The process of recovery after hemiplegia. Stroke 3 (1972), 702—710.

Nicola, G.: The "Rete mirabile" in man. Vasc. Surg. 4 (1970), 156—160.

Nishimoto, A., Takeuchi, S.: Abnormal cerebrovascular network related to the internal carotid arteries. J. Neurosurg. 29 (1968), 255—260.

Nutik, S.: Carotid-anterior cerebral artery anastomosis. Case report. J. Neurosurg. 44 (1976), 378—382.

Obrist, W. D., Thompson, H. D., King, C. H., Wang, H. S.: Determination of regional cerebral blood flow by inhalation of 133 xenon. Circ. Res. 20 (1967), 124—128.

Obrist, W. D., Thompson, M. K., Wang, H. S., Cronquist, S.: A simplified procedure for determining fast compartment rCBF by 133 xenon inhalation. In: R. W. R. Ross Russel: Brain and blood flow, pp. 11—15. London: Pitman. 1971.

Olesen, J.: Cerebral blood flow. Copenhagen: Fadls Forlag. 1974.

Osgood, C. P., Dujovny, M., Maroon, J. C., Janetta, P. J.: Microsurgical mammary-vertebral anastomosis. Second International Symposium on Microneurosurgical Anastomoses for Cerebral Ischemia. Chicago, Illinois (1974).

Osgood, C. P.: Stodged middle cerebral artery embolectomy. J. Surg. Res. 20 (1976), 395—399.

Osgood, P., Dujovny, M., Fleming, M.: Intracranial isolation of the canine circle of Willis. Second International Symposium on Microneurosurgical Anastomoses for Cerebral Ischemia, Chicago, Ill. (1974).

Ostfeld, A. R.: Are strokes reventable? Med. Clin. of Na. 51 (1967), 105—111.

Pauley, J. W., Hughes, J. P.: Giant-cell arteriitis, or arteriitis of the aged. Brit. Med. J. 2 (1960), 1562—1567.

Paulson, G. W., Kapp, J., Cook, W.: Dementia associated with bilateral carotid artery disease. Geriatrics 21 (1960), 159—166.

Peerless, S. J.: Techniques of cerebral revascularization. Clin. Neurosurg. 23 (1976), 258—269.

Piepgras, D. G.: Factors influencing postoperative vascular patency. Clin. Neurosurg. 23 (1976), 310—317.

Piza-Katzer, H.: Mikrochirurgische Technik bei Gefäßen mit einem Durchmesser unter 1,2 mm. Vasa 3 (1974), 293—298.

Planiol, T. H., Pourcelot, L., Pottier, J. M., De Giovanni, E.: Etude de la circulation carotidienne par les méthodes ultrasoniques et la thermographie. Rev. Neurol. *126* (1972), 127—136.

Platzer, W.: Die A. carotis interna im Bereich des Keilbeins bei Primaten. Morph. J. *97* (1956), 220—232.

Platzer, W.: Die Variabilität der A. carotis interna im Sinus cavernosus in Beziehung zur Variabilität der Schädelbasis. Morph. J. *98* (1957), 227—235.

Prosenz, P., Heiss, W. D., Tschabitscher, M., Ehrmann, L.: The value of regional blood flow measurements compared to angiography in the assessment of obstructive neck vessel disease. Stroke *5* (1974), 19—36.

Redondo, A., Le Beau, J.: Traitement des ischémies cérébrales par anastomose artérielle extra-intra-crânienne précoxe. Presented at a meeting of the Société de Neuro-chirurgie de Langue Française, Paris, France, December 1, 1975.

Regli, F.: Die flüchtigen ischämischen zerebralen Attacken. Dtsch. Med. Wschr. *96* (1971), 303—312.

Reichman, O. H., Davis, D. O., Roberts, Th. S., Satovick, R. H.: Anastomosis between STA and cortical branch of MCA for the treatment of occlusive cerebrovascular disease. In: Merei, F. T. (ed.): Reconstructive surgery of brain arteries, pp. 201—218. Budapest: Akadémiai Kiadó. 1974.

Reichman, O. H.: Extracranial-intracranial arterial anastomosis. In: Whisnant, L. P., Sandotz, B. A.: Cerebrovascular diseases (Ninth Conference), pp. 175—186. New York: Grune and Stratton. 1975.

— Continued patency of canine lingual-basilar system. Stroke *3* (1972), 386—591.

— Experimental lingual-basilar arterial micro-anastomosis. J. Neurosurg. *34* (1971), 500—505.

— Complications of cerebral revascularization. Clin. Neurosurg. *23* (1976), 318—335.

— Arteriographic flow patherns following STA-cortical MCA anastomosis. In: Austin, G. H. (ed.): Microneurosurgical anastomoses for cerebral ischemia, pp. 339—358. Springfield, Ill.: Ch. C Thomas. 1976.

Reinstein, L.: All stroke syndrome are not vascular. Arch. Phys. med. Rehabil. *57* (1976), 194—196.

Reisner, H.: Die Karotisinsuffizienz als haemodynamisches und therapeutisches Problem. Wien. klin. Wschr. *78* (1966), 156—160.

— Die neurologische Indikationsstellung zur chirurgischen Behandlung der Carotis interna-Stenosen. Wien. klin. Wschr. *80* (1968), 862—865.

— Die Indikationsstellung zur chirurgischen Therapie des Gehirnschlages. Zeitschr. ärztl. Fortbildg. *65* (1971), 405—409.

— Die Koordinierung klinischer und nichtklinischer Befunde für Diagnostik und Therapie zerebraler Gefäßerkrankungen. Wien. klin. Wschr. *84* (1972), 185—190.

Reisner, H., Felger, G. P., Scherzer, E.: Das weitere Schicksal von 1000 zerebralen Insulten. Wien. klin. Wschr. *73* (1961), 397—402.

Reisner, H., Reisner, Th.: Über traumatisch bedingte zerebrale Gefäßthrombosen. Wien. klin. Wschr. *88* (1976), 158—161.

Rhoton, A. L.: Comparison of flow in arterial and venous graft to basilar artery. Second International Symposium on Microneurosurgical Anastomoses for Cerebral Ischemia. Chicago, Illinois (1974).

Risberg, J., Halsey, J. H., Wills, E. L., Wilson, E. H.: Hemispheric specialization in normal man studied by bilateral measurements of the regional cerebral blood flow. A study with the 133 xe inhalation technique. Brain *98* (1975), 511—524.

Robert, G., Hardy, J.: Problèmes techniques de la microchirurgie vasculaire cérébrale. Neuro-chirurgie (Paris) *19* (1973), 151—164.

Robertson, J. H.: The influence of mechanical factors on the structure of peripheral arteries and the localization of atherosclerosis. J. Clin. Path. *13* (1960), 199—204.

Rockett, J. F.: The radionuclide cerebral angiogram in stroke diagnose. Clin. Neurosurg. (1977), 245—257.

Rogers, L. A.: Microsurgical cerebral anastomosis for the prevention of stroke. N. C. Med. J. *37* (1976), 540—548.

Rosa, M.: Angiotomographic study of the normal cerebral circulation II. The vertebrobasilar system. Neuroradiology *10* (1976), 243—249.

Rosenbaum, Th. J., Sundt, T. M.: Thrombus formation and endothelial alterations in microarterial anastomoses. J. Neurosurg. *47* (1977), 430—441.

Ross Russell, R. W.: Cerebral arterial disease. Edinburgh-London-New York: Churchill Livingstone. 1976.

Rovira, M., Jacas, R., Ley, A.: Collateral circulation in thrombosis of the internal carotid artery and its branches. Acta Radiol. *50* (1958), 101—107.

Ruge, H.: Der Schlaganfall und die fachpädagogische Behandlung seiner Nebenwirkungen bei älteren Patienten mit schwerer Aphasie. Acta Gerontol. *2* (1972), 187—193.

Salazar, J. L.: Intracranial neurosurgical treatment of occlusive cerebrovascular disease. Stroke *7* (1976), 348—353.

Samson, D., Watts, C., Clark, K.: Cerebral revascularization for transient ischemic attacks. Neurology *27* (1977), 767—771.

Scheibert, C. D.: Middle cerebral artery surgery for obstructive lesions. Presented at meeting of Harvey Cushing Society, New Orleans, May 2, 1959.

Schmiedek, P. (ed.): Microsurgery for Stroke. Berlin-Heidelberg-New York: Springer. 1977.

Schmiedek, P., Gratzl, O., Olteanu, V., Steinhoff, H., Baethmann, A., Enzenbach, R.: The contribution of regional cerebral blood flow measurement to the microneurosurgical treatment of cerebral ischemia. International Symposium "Microneurosurgical anastomoses for cerebral ischemia". Loma Linda, California (1973).

Schmiedek, P., Lanksch, W., Olteanu-Nerve, V., Kazner, E., Gratzl, C., Marguth, F.: Combined use of regional cerebral blood flow measurement and computerized tomography for the diagnosis of cerebral ischemia. In: Schmiedek, P. (ed.): Microsurgery for Stroke. Berlin-Heidelberg-New York: Springer. 1977.

Schmiedek, P., Steinhoff, H., Gratzl, O.: Current status of regional cerebral blood flow measurement in revascularisation microsurgery of the brain. Second International Symposium on Microneurosurgical Anastomoses for Cerebral Ischemia. Chicago, Illinois (1974).

Schmiedek, P., Steinhoff, H., Gratzl, O., Steude, U., Enzenbach, R.: rCBF measurements in patients treated for cerebral ischemia by extra-intracranial vascular anastomosis. Europ. Neurol. *6* (1971), 364—368.

Schmiedek, P., Gratzl, O., Spetzler, R., Steinhoff, H., Enzenbach, R., Brendel, W., Marguth, F.: Selection of patients for extra-intracranial arterial bypass surgery based on rCBF measurements. J. Neurosurg. *44* (1976), 303—312.

Schuster, H., Koos, W. Th., Kletter, G.: Quelques particularités de la technique d'anastomose extra-intracrânienne. Neuro-chirurgie (Paris) *22* (1976), 91—96.

——— Some comments on the technique of STA-cortical MCA anastomoses. In: Schmiedek, P. (ed.): Microsurgery for Stroke, pp. 214—217. Berlin-Heidelberg-New York: Springer. 1977.

Shelley, N. Ch.: Embolectomy of middle cerebral artery. J. Neurosurg. *19* (1962), 161—163.

Shillito, J.: Indication for surgery in cerebrovascular accidents. Postgrad. Med. J. *30* (1961), 537—543.

— Strokes in children. Clin. Neurosurg. *23* (1976), 185—219.

Shucart, W. A.: Reopening some occluded carotid arteries. Report of four cases. J. Neurosurg. *45* (1976), 442—446.

Siekert, R. G.: Cerebrovascular survey report for joint council subcommittee on cerebrovascular disease—National Institute Neurological Diseases and Stroke and National Heart and Lung Institute, revised, Rochester, Minn. July 1970, Whiting, Printers and Stationers.

Sindou, M., Brunon, J., Fischer, G., Goutelle, A., Mansuy, L.: L'anastomose extra-intracrânienne préalable à la ligature de la carotide. Neuro-chirurgie (Paris) *23* (1977), 205—213.

Sinzinger, H., Hoyer-Volavsek, Ch., Tschabitscher, M., Perneczky, A.: Alterseinflüsse auf Arterien am Beispiel der Arteria temporalis superficialis. Verh. Anat. Ges. *69* (1975), 885—890.

Skip, J., Garner, J. T.: Reversal of aphasia with superficial temporal artery to middle cerebral artery anastomosis. Surg. Neurol. *5* (1976), 143—145.

Smith, J. W.: Microsurgery: review of the literature and discussion of microtechniques. Plast. reconstr. Surg. *37* (1966), 227—231.

Smith, R., Dalessio, D. J.: Temporal arteriitis.—Why the temporal artery? Headache (1972), 18—19.

Sokoloff, L.: Local cerebral circulation at rest and during altered cerebral activity induced by anestesia or visual stimulation. In: Kety, S. S. (ed.): Regional Neurochemistry. Long Island City: Pergamon. 1961.

Spetzler, R. F., Chater, N. L.: Microvascular arterial bypass in cerebrovascular occlusive disease. In: Koos, W., Böck, F., Spetzler, R. (ed.): Clinical Microneurosurgery, pp. 242—247. Stuttgart: Thieme. 1975.

—— Microvascular bypass surgery. II. Physiological studies. J. Neurosurg. *45* (1976), 508—513.

—— Occipital artery—middle cerebral artery anastomosis for cerebral artery occlusive disease. Surg. Neurol. *2* (1974), 235—238.

Spetzler, R. F., Wing, S. D., Norman, D.: Evaluation of patients with cerebral ischemia using computerized tomography. In: Schmiedek, P. (ed.): Microsurgery for Stroke. Berlin-Heidelberg-New York: Springer. 1977.

Stephens, R. B., Stilwell, D. L.: Arteries and veins of the human brain. Springfield, Ill.: Ch. C Thomas. 1976.

Stephens, H. W.: The Combination of new and old vascular surgical techniques in the aggressive treatment of transient ischemic attacks. Second International Symposium on Microneurosurgical Anastomoses for Cerebral Ischemia. Chicago, Illinois. 1974.

— Microsurgical anastomosis of ten patients at a community hospital. First International Symposium on Microneurosurgical Anastomosis for Cerebral Ischemia, Loma Linda, California, June (1973).

Stephens, R. B., Stilwell, D. L.: Arteries and veins of the human brain. Springfield, Ill.: Ch. C Thomas. 1977.

Sundt, Th. M.: The cerebral autonomic nervous system. A proposed physiologic function and pathophysiologic response in subarachnoid hemorrhage and in focal cerebral ischemia. Mayo Clin. Proc. *48* (1973), 127—137.

Sundt, T. M., Jr.; Stroke: What's new? Cerebral revascularization. Editorial Minn. Med. *59* (1976), 239.

Sundt, T. M., Jr., Siekert, R. G., Piepgras, D. G., Sharbrough, F. W., Houser, O. W.: Bypass surgery for vascular disease of the carotid system. Mayo Clin. Proc. *51* (1976), 677—692.

Suzuki, J., Takaru, A.: Cerebrovascular "moyamoya" disease. Disease showing abnormal net-like vessels in base of brain. Arch. Neurol. *20* (1969), 288—299.

Takeuchi, K.: Occlusive disease of the carotid artery. Recent Adv. in Res. of Nerv. Syst. *5* (1961), 511—513.

Tandler, J.: Zur vergleichenden Anatomie der Kopfarterien bei den Mammalia. Wien: C. Gerold's Sohn. 1899.

— Zur Entwicklungsgeschichte des arteriellen Wundernetzes. Anat. Hefte *94* (1906), 237—265.

Taveras, J. M.: Multiple progressive intracranial arterial occlusion. A syndrome of children and young adults. Amer. J. Roentgenol. *106* (1969), 235—268.

Tew, J. M., Jr.: Reconstructive intracranial vascular surgery for prevention of stroke. Clin. Neurosurg. *22* (1975), 264—280.

Tew, J. M., Jr., Greiner, A. L., Berger, T. S.: Intracranial reconstructive surgery: Indications and operative results. Stroke *8* (1977), 11.

Tew, J. M., Jr., Greiner, A. L., Berger, T. S., Dunsker, S. B., Budde, R. B.: Intracranial vascular bypass: Can it prevent stroke? Mod. Med. *45* (1977), 58—61.

Thompson, J. R., Rouhe, St. A., Austin, G. H., Simmons, Ch.: Angiographic cerebral blood flow patterns in STA-MCA-anastomosis candidates. Second International Symposium on Microneurosurgical Anastomoses for Cerebral Ischemia. Chicago, Illinois. 1974.

Thompson, J. R.: Angiography of brain ischemia and the superficial temporal artery-middle cerebral artery anastomosis candidate. In: Austin, G. M.: Microneurosurgical anastomoses for cerebral ischemia, pp. 157—175. Springfield, Ill.: Ch. C Thomas. 1976.

Torkildsen, A., Koppang, K.: Notes on the collateral cerebral circulation as demonstrated by carotid angiography. J. Neurosurg. *8* (1951), 269—278.

Tönnis, W., Schiefer, W.: Zirkulationsstörungen des Gehirns im Serienangiogramm. Berlin-Göttingen-Heidelberg: Springer. 1959.

Tschabitscher, M., Perneczky, A., Hoyer-Volavsek, Ch., Sinzinger, H.: Untersuchungen über die Gefäßversorgung des Kleinhirns beim Menschen. Verh. Anat. Ges. *69* (1975), 559—561.

Upmark, E., Bickerstaff, E. R.: Vertebral artery occlusion and oral contraceptives. Brit. Med. J. I (1976), 487—488.

Valencak, E., Grunert, V., Mostbeck, A.: Le shunts artério-veineux en physiologie et physio-pathologie cérébrale. Neuro-chirurgie (Paris) *15* (1969), 594—599.

Vollmar, J.: Rekonstruktive Chirurgie der Arterien, pp. 300—345. Stuttgart: G. Thieme. 1975.

— Surgical prevention and therapy of apoplectic stroke. Med. Welt *27* (1976), 844—846.

Waddington, M. H.: The normal anatomy of the middle cerebral artery. In: Austin, G. M.: Microneurosurgical anastomoses for cerebral ischemia, pp. 133—145. Springfield, Ill.: Ch. C Thomas. 1976.

Waltz, A. G.: Pathophysiology of cerebral infarction. Clin. Neurosurg. *23* (1976), 147—154.

— Anatomy and physiology of stroke. Second International Symposium on Microneurosurgical Anastomoses for Cerebral Ischemia. Chicago, Illinois. 1974.

Watts, C.: Cerebral revascularization for stroke. Mod. Med. *73* (1976), 179—181.

Weidner, W., Hanafee, W., Markham, C. E.: Intracranial collateral circulation via leptomeningeal and rete mirabile anastomoses. Neurology *15* (1965), 39—48.

Weinstein, P. R., Chater, N. L., Ausman, J. I., Lamond, R.: Extra-to-intracranial arterial by-pass for occlusive vertebro-basilar cerebrovascular disease. Presented at the 43rd Annual Meeting of the American Association of Neurological Surgeons, Miami Beach, Florida, April 8, 1975.

Weinstein, P. R., Lamond, R., Chater, N. L., Moscow, N.: Anatomical studies of the posterior circulation relevant to possible occipital artery bypass for occipital cerebrovascular disease. Second International Symposium on Microsurgical Anastomoses for Cerebral Ischemia. Chicago, Illinois. 1974.

Welch, K., Stephens, J., Huber, W., Ingersoll, C.: The collateral circulation following middle cerebral branch occlusion. J. Neurosurg. *12* (1955), 361—368.

Welch, K.: Excision of occlusive lesions of the middle cerebral artery. J. Neurosurg. *13* (1956), 73—80.

Wernicke, C.: Lehrbuch der Gehirnkrankheiten, Bd. 83. Kassel-Berlin: Fischer Verlag. 1881.

Whisnant, J., Matsumoto, N., Lila, E.: Transient cerebral ischemic attacks in Rochester, Minnesota. 1945—1969. Mayo Clin. Proc. *48* (1973), 194—198.

Willis, T.: Practice of Physick. London: S. Pordage. 1684.

Woringer, E., Kunlin, J.: Anastomose entre la carotide primitive et la carotide intracrânienne ou la Sylvienne par greffon selon la technique de la suture suspendue. Neuro-chirurgie (Paris) *9* (1963), 181.

World Health Organization: Cerebrovascular disease: prevention, treatment and rehabilitation. Report of a WHO meeting. Who Technical Series 469. 1971.

Wright, J.: The microscopical appearences of human peripheral arteries during growth and aging. J. Clin. Path. *16* (1963), 499—522.

Wright, L.: Experimental cerebral ischemia. Angiology *16* (1965), 397—404.

Wylie, E. J., Hein, M. F., Adams, J. E.: Intracranial hemorrhage following revascularization for treatment of acute stroke. J. Neurosurg. *21* (1964), 212—215.

Yaşargil, M. G.: Experimental small vessel surgery in dog including patching and grafting of cerebral vessels and the formation of functional extra-intracranial shunts. In: Donaghy, R. M. P., Yaşargil, M. G.: Micro-vascular surgery, pp. 87—126. St. Louis: C. V. Mosby Co. 1967.

Yaşargil, M. G., Yonekawa, Y.: Brain vascularization by intracranially transpanted omentum. Second International Symposium on Microneurosurgical Anastomoses for Cerebral Ischemia. Chicago, Illinois. 1974.

— — Results of microsurgical extra-intracranial arterial bypass in the treatment of cerebral ischemia. Neurosurgery *1* (1977), 22—24.

Yaşargil, M. G.: Mikrotechnische Behandlung der Hirnarterien-Verschlüsse. In: Duchosal, P. W., Krähenbühl, B.: Akute zerebrale Durchblutungsstörungen, pp. 78—98. Bern: H. Huber. 1976.

— Microsurgical approach to the cerebrovascular diseases. In: Fusek, J., Kunce, Z.: Present Limits of Neurosurgery, Avicenum. 1972.

Yaşargil, M. G., Krayenbühl, H. A., Jacobson, J. H.: Microneurosurgical arterial reconstruction. Surgery *67* (1970), 221—233.

Yaşargil, M. G.: Microsurgery applied to neurosurgery. Stuttgart: G. Thieme. 1969.

Yonekawa, Y., Yaşargil, M. G.: Extra-intracranial arterial anastomosis: clinical and technical aspects results. Advances and Technical Standards in Neurosurgery, Vol. 3, pp. 47—78. Wien-New York: Springer. 1976.

Ziegler, D. K., Hassanein, R. S.: Prognosis in patients with TIA's. Stroke *4* (1973), 666—673.

Zlotnik, E. I.: Thrombectomy of the middle cerebral artery. J. Neurosurg. *42* (1975), 723—725.

Zumstein, B.: Personal communication, 1975.

Subject Index